(

n

the late

oplication, .
the barcoc

Date D

Legionella Infections

Legionella Infections

Christopher L.R. Bartlett MSc, MB, FFCM

Consultant Epidemiologist
PHLS Communicable Disease Surveillance Centre
London and
Honorary Lecturer
Department of Environmental and Preventive Medicine
The Medical College of St Bartholomew's Hospital
London

Alastair D. Macrae MD, FRCPath, DipBact

Formerly of Public Health Laboratory Service
Nottingham

John T. Macfarlane MA, DM(Oxon), MRCP

Consultant Physician
City Hospital
Nottingham and
Clinical Teacher
University of Nottingham

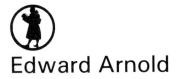

Edward Arnold

First published in Great Britain 1986 by
Edward Arnold (Publishers) Ltd, 41 Bedford Square, London WC1B 3DQ

Edward Arnold (Australia) Pty Ltd, 80 Waverley Road, Caulfield East,
Victoria 3145, Australia

Edward Arnold , 3 East Read Street, Baltimore, Maryland 21202, USA

British Library Cataloguing in Publication Data

Bartlett, C.L.R.
  Legionella infections.
  1. Legionnaires' disease
  I. Title II. Macrae, Alastair D.
  III. Macfarlane, John T.
  616.2′41   RC152.7

ISBN 0-7131-4506-4

Whilst the advice and information in this book is believed to be true and accurate
at the date of going to press, neither the authors nor the publisher can accept any
legal responsibility or liability for any errors or omissions that may be made.

Text set in 10/11pt Times Compugraphic
by Colset Private Limited, Singapore
Printed and bound in Great Britain by Butler & Tanner Ltd, Frome and London

Preface

The dramatic events which followed the Pennsylvania State Convention of the American Legion in Philadelphia in July 1976 unveiled a previously unrecognized form of acute lobar pneumonia which consequently was named legionnaires' disease. The illness developed mainly in elderly individuals after an incubation period of about 2–10 days. Mortality was high. There was no evidence of person-to-person spread and transmission appeared to be by inhalation of an agent from a common environmental source. After prolonged and intensive laboratory studies the disease was found to be due to a new family of organisms later named the Legionellaceae with *Legionella pneumophila* as the first species. The interest aroused, resulted in a widening search in many countries both for the disease and the organisms; the First International Symposium devoted to its study was held in Atlanta, Georgia, USA some 2 years later and this in turn gave fresh impetus to investigation.

The disease, found whenever searches were made, presented in various guises ranging from the classical primary lobar pneumonia to milder or non-pneumonic forms. It occurred both as sporadic infections and in outbreaks which were often associated with hospitals and hotels. Retrospective investigations revealed and clarified several earlier and previously unrecognized outbreaks of the disease.

As cultural techniques improved and became more widely known, the number of additions to the new family of Legionellaceae from patient material and from environmental sources, escalated. A Second International Symposium was held in 1983 at which much new information was presented on the various species of legionella and their identification as well as the epidemiology of infections including sources and mode of transmission. At least 11 serogroups of *L. pneumophila* and 22 other species of Legionellaceae have been described. Legionella infections have been recognized in all continents and outbreaks have been reported from several countries.

This book describes the present knowledge of the clinical picture, pathology, treatment and epidemiology of the disease, the characteristics and habitats of the family of Legionellaceae are described, potential sources of infection identified and methods of control and prevention discussed. Epidemiology is dealt with in Chapter 3 where it is relevant to clinical practice and in Chapters 7 and 8 in relation to the investigation and control of sources of infection. Each chapter has been written, as far as possible, to stand on its own for easy reference. This has inevitably led to some repetition but we have tried to keep this to a minimum.

1986

C.L.R.B
A.D.M
J.T.M

Acknowledgements

We are indebted to Dr N.S. Galbraith, Sir Robert Williams, Dr S.R. Palmer, Dr B.D.W. Harrison, Dr A.E. Wright, Mr P.J.L. Dennis and Dr P. Appleby for their valuable comments on various chapters of the manuscript. We wish to acknowledge our colleagues, particularly those within the Public Health Laboratory Service, who have contributed to our knowledge of the subject.

Finally we wish to thank Dr F.G. Rodgers for providing the electron micrographs, Dr A.D. Pearson for two photographs of cooling towers, Dr J.S.P. Jones for photographs of pathological changes, Dr G. Brundrett for a photograph and one of the figures, Mr R. Edwards for the GLC profiles, Miss Penny Forsyth who prepared the other figures and Miss Nina Burghiner for her untiring efforts in typing and proof reading the manuscript.

Contents

1 The Family Legionellaceae

Following the outbreak of pneumonia which occurred after the 1976 American Legion State Convention in Philadelphia, studies of lung tissue from four of the fatal cases eventually yielded a small, previously uniden- tified, Gram-negative organism which at first became known as the legionnaires' disease (LD) bacterium (McDade *et al.*, 1977). This isolation resulted from guinea-pig intraperitoneal inoculation followed by transfer of infectious extracts to the yolk sac of the developing chick embryo. Such a technique, commonly used in rickettsia investigations, had been applied because rickettsias were included among the possible causative agents of the outbreak. The organism, not being a rickettsia which typically grows only intracellularly, was then subcultured from yolk sac suspension. Of those media tried, only a modified Mueller–Hinton agar containing IsoVitalex and haemoglobin (MH-IH) was found suitable. This medium had previously been used successfully for other organisms not readily adaptable to routine bacteriological media (Feeley *et al.*, 1978).

About the same time a Gram-negative bacterium was cultured directly from the pleural fluid and lung tissue of a fatal case of pneumonia at Flint, Michigan. Grown on a commercially available enriched chocolate agar medium it was found to resemble closely the legionnaires' disease bacterium (Dumoff, 1979). These organisms were small rods, oxidase and catalase posi- tive, and did not reduce nitrates, degrade urea or use carbohydrates. They were fastidious in their growth requirements, aerobic, with a narrow optimal pH and temperature range and had a deoxyribonucleic acid (DNA) guanine plus cytosine content of 39 mol per cent (Brenner *et al.*, 1979). This content was later modified to range between 38 and 52 mol per cent (Brenner *et al.*, 1985).

Checks of other similar, though unclassified organisms isolated in previous years, unearthed two other strains resembling the Philadelphia bac- terium. One had come from the sudden short outbreak of febrile disease among staff and visitors at the County Health Department, Pontiac, Michigan in 1968. Now classed as the Pontiac strain, it was identified in 1977 after its recovery from the stored frozen lung tissue of guinea-pigs. These animals had been placed in various parts of the departmental building after the outbreak, to allow exposure to aerosols from the evaporative condenser cooling water of the air-conditioning system. The strain was also recovered from the cooling water itself (Glick *et al.*, 1978; Kaufmann *et al.*, 1981). The other, named Olda, had been isolated by guinea-pig and yolk sac inoculation in 1947 from the blood of a patient with a febrile respiratory illness of suspected rickettsial origin. Unclassified for 30 years, it had been regarded as guinea-pig derived, possibly a rickettsia, and unrelated to the patient's illness until its correct identity was finally established (McDade *et al.*, 1979).

The role of the legionnaires' bacterium in the Philadelphia outbreak was confirmed by its isolation from consolidated lung tissue of fatal cases and the demonstration of a humoral immune response to it in survivors. Since then, it has been implicated in numerous other outbreaks, including hospital acquired (nosocomial) and sporadic infections. It has also emerged that there is a large family of these organisms widely distributed in natural and artificial water sources. The family includes an increasing number of distinct species, some containing multiple serogroups (see Table 1.1). Though not always a cause of illness, more and more of these species have been found in certain circumstances to become opportunistic pathogens causing pneumonia or milder infections.

The first classification of the organism, together with the name *Legionella pneumophila* – from the Greek *pneumo* for lung and *philos* for loving – genus *Novum*, species *nova* of the family Legionellaceae was introduced at the First International Symposium on legionnaires' disease, Atlanta, USA in November 1978. The Philadelphia 1 strain isolated from lung tissue became the type strain (Brenner *et al.*, 1979). This confirmation of the organism as a distinct species marked the culmination of some two years' study of its characteristics which had included growth, morphology, biochemical reactions, fatty acid content and DNA homology. The later emergence of more than one species had enlarged the new genus, and the unrelatedness of this genus to other organisms, the new family. Names of the then known legionella species were included in the International Committee on Systematic Bacteriology Approved Lists of Bacterial Names. Based on certain phenotypic characteristics and DNA relatedness two new genera, *Fluoribacter*, comprising *L. bozemanii*, *L. dumoffii* and *L. gormanii*, and *Tatlockia* comprising *L. micdadei* and related organisms were promulgated (Report, 1981). Doubts were later expressed over the usefulness of this step and its justification (Brenner *et al.*, 1982) and with so much common ground among the species it would seem preferable at this stage to persist with a one-genus family of Legionellaceae (Brenner, 1984; Brenner *et al.*, 1985).

Known species of legionella have been listed in Table 1.1. *L. pneumophila* possesses at least eleven serogroups, though as a cause of human illness serogroup 1 has predominated. Among other species, 22 have been named so far with *L. bozemanii*, *L. longbeachae*, *L. feeleii* and *L. hackeliae* each possessing two serogroups; further additions await classification (Bercovier *et al.*, 1986; Brenner, 1984; Brenner *et al.*, 1985; Brown *et al.*, 1984; Gorman *et al.*, 1985; Thacker *et al.*, 1985a,b, 1986). Distinctive features which characterize this family of organisms are now discussed.

Table 1.1 Legionella species

Legionella pneumophila	serogroups 1–11	Legionella anisa	
″ bozemanii	serogroups 1 and 2	″ maceachernii	
″ dumoffii		″ jamestowniensis	
″ gormanii		″ rubrilucens	
″ micdadei		″ erythra	
″ longbeachae	serogroups 1 and 2	″ spiritensis	
″ jordanis		″ parisiensis	
″ oakridgensis		″ cherrii	
″ wadsworthii		″ steigerwaltii	
″ feeleii	serogroups 1 and 2	″ santicrusis	
″ sainthelensi		″ israelensis	
″ hackeliae	serogroups 1 and 2		

Morphology, structure and composition

By utilizing negative stain electron microscopy on organisms in infected lung tissue, legionella species have appeared as mainly small coccobacilli measuring up to 0.5 μm by 1–3 μm, with occasional longer forms of 10–15 μm or more. The longer organisms became more evident after subculture. Division takes place by pinching septate fission within the outer lamella of the bacterial membrane (Rodgers, 1979). The organisms possess smooth, fine-grained or irregularly convoluted surfaces, sometimes vacuolated with sudanophilic inclusions and non-parallel sides tapering to rounded ends. They are non-sporing, non-acid-fast, Gram-negative organisms. However, counter staining is poor unless the staining time is prolonged or dilute carbol fuchsin is applied. This feature may be connected with their unusual fatty acid composition. Particularly when cultured on suboptimal solid agar medium, as was the experience with initial isolates, filamentous growth with organisms up to 50 μm in length have been found.

Specific identification of organisms is still based largely on fluorescent antibody staining methods (Cherry *et al.*, 1978) with the development of monoclonal antibodies an additional factor. This has, on the one hand, provided a species-specific *L. pneumophila* reagent, diagnostically useful (Edelstein *et al.*, 1985; Gosting *et al.*, 1984; Tenover *et al.*, 1985). On the other hand, the use of antibody panels, highlighting strain differences has led to the identification of major and minor subgroups particularly of *L. pneumophila* serogroup 1, thus helping to identify sources of outbreaks.

Joly and Winn (1984) used mouse monoclonal antibodies to label their *L. pneumophila* serogroup 1 subgroups A, B and C according to staining pattern. Watkins, Tobin and colleagues (1985) also depicted three major subgroups for this serogroup and named these after representative strains Pontiac 1, Olda and Bellingham 1. To avoid future confusion an international subclassification scheme based on 10 major subgroups has been put forward (Joly *et al.*, 1986).

Other techniques for identification have included slide agglutination or coagglutination (Groothuis *et al.*, 1984; Thacker *et al.*, 1985a, 1986; Wilkinson and Fikes, 1981), immunoferritin staining in electron microscopy (Rodgers and Macrae, 1979) and specific DNA probes (Grimont *et al.*, 1985).

Legionella soluble antigens found in serum and urine have been detected by tests such as radioimmunoassay, latex agglutination or ELISA (Kohler *et al.*, 1984). Other useful, though non-specific stains, include Giemsa and Gimenez applied to organisms both in smears and tissues and silver impregnation e.g. Dieterle or a modification of Warthin-Starry (Faine, 1965) in tissues. Immunoperoxidase staining has also been described (Boyd and McWilliams, 1982).

Their presence in water had suggested that the legionella species were likely to be motile. Confirmation of this came from reports of flagella seen by light and immunofluorescence microscopy (Thomason *et al.*, 1979). Electron microscopic observation showed the flagella to be polar or subpolar, mainly single but occasionally paired, up to 8 μm in length and 14–20 nm in diameter. As with other Gram-negative bacteria they were linked to the cell wall of the organism through a basal body or granule comprising a hook-like structure. Additionally, the fimbriae or pili, distributed evenly around the bacterial surface were observed during the logarithmic phase of growth but tended to disappear later (Rodgers *et al.*, 1980). Similar findings were reported from the United States (Chandler *et al.*, 1980a). These authors also noted flagella on legionella species other than *L. pneumophila*. Investigations of infected human lung tissue also revealed flagella on some extracellular organisms in alveolar spaces (Chandler *et al.*, 1980b).

Thin section electron microscopy of organisms, showed that legionella species possess the same prokaryotic structure detail as other small Gram-negative bacteria, having a thin-walled double cell envelope and ribosome and dispersed nuclear material in the cytoplasm (Rodgers, 1979). The outer envelope layer appeared electron dense, loose and undulating, the inner cytoplasmic layer less dense. Between these was a discontinuous layer for which the evidence, including the detection of diaminopimelic acid (Guerrant *et al.*, 1979), suggests that it contains a peptidoglycan band (Rodgers and Davey, 1982; Hébert *et al.*, 1984). No surrounding mucopolysaccharide layer was detectable on staining organisms with ruthenium red (Rodgers, 1979) but such a layer was demonstrated on some low-passage organisms from four legionella species (Hébert *et al.*, 1984) a factor which may have some bearing on pathogenicity.

The legionella species are unusual for Gram-negative bacteria in their distinctive lipid composition. They have a high phospholipid content including phosphatidylcholine in their cell envelopes (Hindahl and Iglewski, 1984) and branched chain fatty acids make up 80–90 per cent of the total cellular fatty acid content (Finnerty *et al.*, 1979; Moss *et al.*, 1981). Analysis of these acids by gas–liquid chromatography and mass spectrometry has revealed a number of characteristic profiles for different legionella species (Cherry *et al.*, 1982). By comparing four fatty acid peaks, Edwards and Feltham (1983) distinguished three groups of legionella and found also that these organisms were taxonomically distinct from a number of other Gram-negative species investigated. For *L. pneumophila* the major acid component is iso-16:0 with lesser amounts of other acids namely iso-14:0, anti iso-15:0, iso-16:1 and anti iso-17:0. Legionella species also possess ubiquinones (coenzyme Q) with long isoprenoid side-chains sited in the bacterial plasma membranes (Collins and Gilbart, 1983; Hoffman, 1984; Karr *et al.*, 1982). Variation in the number of isoprene units can be of use as chemotaxonomic markers in distinguishing between species and aiding classification through the use of high performance liquid chromatographic analysis (Gilbart and Collins, 1985).

Other features utilized in the classification of legionella species include:

(i) Estimation of their nucleic acid guanine plus cytosine content which has to be of the order of 39 mol per cent but may range between 38 and 52 mol per cent.

(ii) A genome size of 2.5×10^9 daltons.

(iii) Deoxyribonucleic acid (DNA) relatedness. To be members of a particular species, organisms must show a greater than 70 per cent relatedness to the species type strain and to each other in hybridization studies with extracts of their DNA. Dissimilar species will not show this. (Brenner, 1984; Brenner *et al.*, 1979; Brenner *et al.*, 1985.)

Cultivation of Legionellaceae

The original member of the family Legionellaceae, *L. pneumophila*, described as a fastidious, slow-growing aerobic, Gram-negative bacterium, was recovered by the now well publicized technique of guinea-pig and egg yolk sac inoculation (McDade *et al.*, 1977). Other early strains representative of various legionella species were similarly isolated. The guinea-pig technique succeeded when sufficient numbers of virulent organisms, from both human infections and environmental sources, were injected intraperitoneally. Pyrexial, often fatal, illness resulted, with fibrinopurulent peritonitis containing many organisms in exudates. Other organs, including lung, could also be affected, with necrotic suppurative foci present, though the characteristic pneumonia observed in man did not develop (Chandler *et al.*, 1979). Attempts to induce this by aerosol inhalation were at first unsuccessful (Berendt *et al.*, 1980) until the use of fine aerosol droplets less than 5 μm in size containing infectious organisms made it possible (Baskerville *et al.*, 1981). Strains of lesser virulence, including organisms after passage on bacteriological media, cause minor or no illness though they can multiply in the tissues and stimulate an antibody response.

After the initial isolation in guinea-pigs, legionella organisms were adapted to or even directly cultured on bacteriological media. The first successful solid medium, supplemented Mueller–Hinton (MH-IH) agar, led to the finding that growth of legionella was governed by the presence of L-cysteine hydrochloride and a soluble form of iron such as ferric pyrophosphate. These substances have become components of the solid and liquid media now in use. This discovery resulted in the introduction of a new clear medium, Feeley–Gorman (F-G) agar, which gave improved growth, permitted brown pigment formation and production of fluorescence in the presence of long wave ultraviolet light (Feeley *et al.*, 1978). Further development introduced the charcoal yeast extract (CYE) agar medium considered sufficiently sensitive to initiate growth from an inoculum of about 100 viable organisms in a 50 μl volume and able to produce readily visible colonies within 48–72 hours (Feeley *et al.*, 1979). Modification of the CYE medium by incorporating

N-2-acetamido-2-amino-ethanesulfonic acid (ACES) buffer and α-keto-glutarate followed. This aided legionella growth as did the inclusion of a range of antimicrobial substances to suppress other organisms (Edelstein, 1981). Further additions have included glycine, useful when sampling environmental sources (Wadowsky and Yee, 1981) and dyes such as bromo-cresol purple and bromothymol blue (Vickers *et al.*, 1981) or aniline blue (Holmes, 1982) to differentiate between species.

In the course of early legionella studies a blood agar medium enriched with L-cysteine and soluble iron salts was found capable of producing readily visible colonies 2–3 mm in diameter after 48–72 hours' incubation both with laboratory adapted strains and direct lung isolates (Greaves, 1980). During searches for legionella in water systems of hotels and hospitals, CYE agar and enriched blood agar (EBA) gave comparable results (Dennis *et al.*, 1981). However, it was noted that the presence of sodium chloride in the EBA medium had an inhibitory effect unless a pH of 6.9 was maintained. Replacement of the sodium chloride by potassium phosphate buffer pH7 markedly improved its performance. In a further comparison (Dennis *et al.*, 1982) the improved CYE medium (Edelstein, 1981) and the now designated legionella blood agar (LBA) medium were of similar sensitivity. However, Keathley and Winn (1984) found the Greaves' medium less effective than CYE agar but had used only the original formula. In most diagnostic laboratories the CYE medium is now used.

Various liquid media for legionella culture, antigen production and anti-biotic assays have been described of which the filter-sterilized buffered yeast extract broth (Johnson *et al.*, 1982) with added α-ketoglutarate (Barbaree *et al.*, 1983) is probably the most useful. The presence of blood-borne organisms has supported an early bacteraemic phase in legionellosis since guinea-pig inoculation provided the Tatlock strain of *L. micdadei* in 1943 (Hébert *et al.*, 1980) and the Olda strain of *L. pneumophila* in 1947 (McDade *et al.*, 1979). The use of liquid media for direct isolation provided further evidence (Edelstein *et al.*, 1979; Macrae *et al.*, 1979).

Blood culture should thus be part of the investigations at the onset of respiratory illness with subculture to solid legionella medium when the disease is suspected (Chester *et al.*, 1983; Martin *et al.*, 1984; Rihs *et al.*, 1985).

Ecology

Under laboratory conditions legionella species behave as fastidious organisms, yet their natural presence in aquatic habitats (see Appendix) indicates a considerable capacity for survival. Some explanation for this ability has emerged from the finding of *L. pneumophila* in mats of blue-green algae containing *Fischerella* species of cyanobacterium, which were growing in thermal effluents at 45° at a pH between 6.9 and 7.6 (Tison *et al.*, 1980). It was thought that release of organic substrates from active photosynthesis could provide a nutritive base for legionella multiplication. Satellite growth in the presence of a strain of *Flavobacterium breve* has also been reported (Wadowsky and Yee, 1983). Multiplication of *L. pneumophila* in naturally contaminated waters may be enhanced by the presence of various compounds and constituents of rubber and retarded by other substances such as thiuram, facts which are important in relation to plumbing installations in large buildings (Colbourne *et al.*, 1984; Colbourne and Ashworth, 1986; Niedeveld *et al.*, 1986). Studies using model hot water distribution systems have shown that *L. pneumophila* will readily establish itself in a biofilm on different types of surfaces and materials (Schofield and Locci, 1985a, b; Schofield and Wright, 1984).

L. pneumophila is present in lung intra-alveolar macrophages during human infection either from phagocytosis or the result of engulfment followed by intracellular multiplication. It has also been shown, after attachment, to replicate within the cytoplasm of cell cultures including human embryonic lung fibroblasts and continuous lines of Vero and HEp2 cells. Eventual destruction and lysis of cells with bacterial release ensues (Rodgers and Oldham, 1984; Wong *et al.*, 1980); this effect, coupled with a release of toxic products may help to explain the marked pulmonary necrosis which occurs during a pneumonic attack leading sometimes to abscess formation (Winn and Myerowitz, 1981). Similarly, it has been suggested (Anand *et al.*, 1983; Holden *et al.*, 1984; Rowbotham, 1980) that legionella survival in aqueous natural habitats may be related to their capacity to invade and multiply in free-living amoebae of the *Acanthamoeba* and *Naegleria* species and in certain protozoa (Fields *et al.*, 1984).

Metabolism and toxicity

The energy requirements and characteristics of the legionella species support the view that they constitute a distinct taxonomic group with unusual metabolism. These organisms do not ferment commonly utilized carbohydrates, but make use of amino acids for energy and carbon. They are catalase positive, proteolytic, and hydrolyse gelatin, but do not reduce urea or nitrate. Cysteine is necessary for growth but in the case of *L. pneumophila* and probably other species, a lack of the enzymes serine transacetylase and o-acetylserine sulfhydrylase prevents its intrinsic formation (Hoffman, 1984). Known exceptions to this are the species *L. oakridgensis* and *L. jordanis* which do not require added cysteine when passaged. Despite some lack of uniformity, other amino acids such as arginine, isoleucine, leucine, methionine, phenylalanine or tyrosine, proline, serine, threonine and valine have a role in supporting growth. Though legionella do not necessarily need more iron than other bacteria, soluble iron can have a stimulatory effect (George *et al.*, 1980) and increased plasma iron if present in the elderly may be related to more severe disease (Quinn and Weinberg, 1984). In plasma, ordinarily there are inadequate amounts of the free ionic iron needed for bacterial growth, due to the presence of iron binding proteins such as transferrin and lactoferrin. Such substances, being only partly iron-saturated will immediately take up newly released ions but should an excess of iron become available to enable uptake by bacteria, multiplication can proceed. On the other hand, even when the iron available is minimal, pathogenic organisms, including some from Gram-negative species, are able to code for and therefore produce iron-chelating substances such as enterochelin and aerobactin. These compete for the available iron and transport it to bacterial surface receptors. This bypassing of a defensive mechanism enables bacterial multiplication and invasion of the tissues to take place (Bullen, 1985). Whether any such additional proteins, if present in bacterial outer membranes, could provide markers of pathogenicity is at present uncertain.

The main distinguishing features have been established though it is clear that as isolates increase minor inconsistences of characterization become apparent. The brown pigment which surrounds legionella colonies grown on transparent yeast extract agar medium containing L-tyrosine is thought to be a melanin compound activated by bacterial tyrosinase (Baine and Rasheed, 1979). This can help to distinguish most legionella species from other organisms though it is not produced by *L. micdadei* or *L. wadsworthii*. Most species produce beta-lactamase but *L. micdadei*, *L. feeleii* and *L. maceachernii* are exceptions, a feature which may have a bearing on treatment. Hippurate hydrolysis may help to distinguish *L. pneumophila* and *L. feeleii* from others though not all strains do this. After the addition of dyes such as bromocresol purple and bromothymol blue to buffered CYE agar, *L. pneumophila* produces large, flat white to pale green colonies, *L. bozemanii*, *L. dumoffii* and *L. gormanii* small, convex, distinct greenish shiny colonies and *L. micdadei* small, round, blue-grey colonies (Brenner, 1984; Vickers *et al.*, 1981). A system for identifying legionellas from these characteristics has been put forward (Vickers and Yu, 1984).

Though early attempts to associate the severity of legionella pneumonia with bacterial endotoxin did not succeed in identifying a specific toxic lipopolysaccharide, it is now becoming apparent that several bacterial components may play a synergistic role in both pathogenesis and immunity (Wong and Feeley, 1983). Surface antigens providing serogroup specificity can have endotoxic properties and experimentally can cause pyrogenicity, weight-loss, skin reactions and sometimes death. They can also function as adjuvants by stimulating particularly, delayed hypersensitivity as well as antibody booster response. Proteolytic activity by the organisms has been reported (Müller, 1984). Protein exotoxins of low molecular weight, possibly interrelated, have been extracted from bacterial culture filtrates or from acidified extracts of sonnicated bacterial cells. They are lethal to mice, chick embryos and cultured cells including macrophages, interfering with host cell oxidative metabolism and suppressing phagocytosis (Wong and Feeley, 1983). Proteases may share in the induction of lung lesions (Conlan *et al.*, 1986).

Studies of the enzymatic activities of Legionellaceae can distinguish this group from other organisms though within the group profiles were homogenous (Nolte *et al.*, 1982). Among extracellular enzymes with cytotoxic and cytolytic properties are haemolysins (Thorpe and Miller, 1984). Cytolysis may be related to phospholipase C activity (Baine, 1985).

Plasmids have a capacity to transfer between organisms not only of similar but of differing bacterial species, a factor which may affect the pathogenic potential of recipients. They have been found in both clinical and environmental isolates of legionellas though more often in the latter (Brown *et al.*, 1982; Mather *et al.*, 1983). Transfer of plasmids from *Escherichia coli* to legionella has been accomplished (Chen *et al.*, 1984). Plasmid DNA has not, so far, been correlated with any adverse phenotypic traits among these organisms (Aye *et al.*, 1981; Hoffman, 1984). Plasmid and peptide analysis, by providing an additional means of distinguishing strains from different sources is useful epidemiologically in the study of outbreaks (Brown *et al.*, 1985). Comparison of organisms from epidemic and endemic sources by multilocus enzyme electrophoresis, typing with monoclonal antibodies and plasmid analysis may allow separation of those strains causing disease from others and aid in the selection of sites for disinfection (Edelstein *et al.*, 1986).

Pathogenicity and immunity

Legionella species are found in aqueous habitats in which they appear readily able to multiply extracellularly. Human infection is a relatively unusual chance phenomenon. The circumstances which lead up to this are still not entirely clear though factors such as the virulence and dosage of the infecting organisms and the susceptibility of the host are relevant. Human-to-human spread is unusual or non-existent.

To be pathogenic the living organisms, as facultative intracellular parasites, have to make contact with engulfing cells such as macrophages in the lung alveoli. This occurs after the inhalation of small aerosol particles which contain viable bacteria in a phase of multiplication. The bacteria must attach to the surfaces of susceptible cells by a process of adhesion from either physical or chemical attraction. They may be assisted in this by their motility due to flagella and pili. Once drawn within the cell cytoplasm by cellular microvilli and filopodia (Rodgers and Oldham, 1984) they may be destroyed by the body's defensive processes. More often they overcome these by releasing secretory enzymes or toxins and proceed to multiply intracellularly. Destruction of the host cell follows with release of bacteria, toxic products and further cellular invasion. The lung is the main organ showing pathological damage, though spread to other parts of the body can occur, evidenced by bacteraemia and by the appearance of soluble serogroup antigen in serum and urine (Bibb *et al.*, 1984). This supports the hypothesis that bacterial toxins can account for fever and other manifestations during the illness.

In non-pneumonic illness, organisms may be unable to penetrate as far as the lung because the bacterially charged aerosol droplets are too large. An alternative hypothesis is that the organisms are non-viable but may still release potent endo and exotoxins sufficient to induce illness. A further possibility is that certain variants, may lack virulence. Such a change has been observed after subculture of strains on bacteriological media (Bornstein *et al.*, 1984). Strains of the same serogroup, though from different sources or outbreaks, may belong to different subgroups as demonstrated by restriction endonuclease analysis (Ketel *et al.*, 1984), gel electrophoresis and monoclonal antibodies (Bissett *et al.*, 1984; Joly *et al.*, 1986; Watkins *et al.*, 1985).

Legionella infections result in the development of humoral and cell mediated immunity. Circulating antibody in the form of immunoglobulins M, G and less commonly A usually reaches its peak during convalescence. It is mainly a serogroup-specific reaction to the bacterial surface antigen and is relatively long-lasting. It may be accompanied by short-lived cross-reactions with other serogroups or species due to release of common antigens from the process of bacterial disruption. This humoral antibody may be passively transferred but, by itself, does not have a completely protective effect against virulent organisms. In combination with complement it aids phagocytosis of the relevant legionella species by polymorphonuclear leucocytes and monocytes or macrophages. However this does relatively little to impede intracellular multiplication so that its role has limitations.

Experimentally, monocytes incubated with lymphocytes in the presence of the mitogen concanavalin A can reduce the phagocytosis of *L. pneumophila* and slow its intracellular multiplication (Horwitz, 1984). This cell-mediated effect will also appear when cell-free extracts or cytokines from concanavalin A-treated monocyte cell cultures are used. Likewise, monocytes from convalescent legionnaires' disease patients will react in the presence of lymphocytes to produce cytokines specifically able to reduce *L. pneumophila* intracellular multiplication. In combination with specific antibody and complement the organisms will be killed. This supports the view that cell-mediated immunity has its role in the host defence against legionella infection.

References

Anand, C.M., Skinner, A.R., Malic, A. *et al.* (1983). Interaction of *L. pneumophila* and a free living amoeba. (Acanthamoeba palestinensis). *J. Hyg Camb* **91**, 167–78.

Aye, T., Wachsmuth, K., Feeley, J.C. *et al.* (1981). Plasmid profiles of *Legionella* species. *Curr Microbiol* **6**, 389–94.

Baine, W.B. (1985). Cytolytic and phospholipase C activity in *Legionella* species. *J Gen Microbiol* **131**, 1383–91.

Baine, W.B. and Rasheed, J.K. (1979). Aromatic substrate specificity of browning by cultures of the Legionnaires' disease bacterium. *Ann Intern Med* **90**, 619–20.

Barbaree J.M., Sanchez, A. and Sanden, G. (1983). Tolerance of Legionella species to sodium chloride. *Curr Microbiol* **9**, 1–5.

Baskerville, A., Fitzgeorge, R.B., Broster, M. *et al.* (1981). Experimental transmission of Legionnaires' disease by exposure to aerosols of *Legionella pneumophila*. *Lancet* **2**, 1389–90.

Bercovier, H., Steigerwalt, A.G., Derhi-Cochin, M. *et al.* (1986). Isolation of legionellae from oxidation ponds and fishponds in Israel and description of *Legionella israelensis* sp. nov. *Int J Syst Bact* **36**, 368–71.

Berendt, R.F., Young, H.W., Allen, R.G. and Knutsen, G.L. (1980). Dose-response of guinea-pigs experimentally infected with aerosols of *Legionella pneumophila*. *J Infect Dis* **141**, 186–92.

Bibb, W.F., Arnow, P.M., Thacker, L. and McKinney, R.M. (1984). Detection of soluble *Legionella pneumophila* antigens in serum and urine specimens by enzyme-linked immunosorbent assay with monoclonal and polyclonal antibodies. *J Clin Microbiol* **20**, 478–82.

Bissett, M., Nygaard, G., Lee, J. *et al.* (1984). Polyacrilamide gel electrophoresis in the characterization of unusual *Legionella pneumophila* strains isolated from patients in a San Francisco hospital. In *Legionella: Proceedings of the 2nd International Symposium: Washington, DC.*, pp. 86–9. Edited by Thornsberry, C., Balows, A., Feeley, J.C. and Jakubowski, W. American Society for Microbiology, Washington.

Bornstein, N., Nowicki, M. and Fleurette, J. (1984). Loss of virulence of *Legionella pneumophila* serogroup 1 with conversion of cells to long filamentous rods. In *Legionella: Proceedings of the 2nd International Symposium: Washington, DC.*, pp. 70-71. Edited by Thornsberry, C., Balows, A., Feeley, J.C. and Jakubowski, W. American Society of Microbiology, Washington.

Boyd, J.F. and McWilliams, E. (1982). Immunoperoxidase staining of *Legionella pneumophila. Histopathology* **6**, 191-6.

Brenner, D.J. (1984). Classification of Legionellae. In *Legionella: Proceedings of the 2nd International Symposium: Washington, DC.*, pp. 55-60. Edited by Thornsberry, C., Balows, A., Feeley, J.C. and Jakubowski, W. American Society for Microbiology, Washington.

Brenner, D.J., Feeley, J.C. and Feldman, R.A. (1982). Confusion in bacterial nomenclature. *ASM News* **48**, 511-12.

Brenner, D.J., Steigerwalt, A.G. and McDade, J.E. (1979). Classification of the Legionnaires' disease bacterium: *Legionella pneumophila*, genus novum, species nova, of the Family Legionellaceae, familia nova. *Ann Intern Med* **90**, 656-8.

Brenner, D.J., Steigerwalt, A.G., Gorman, G.W. *et al.* (1985). Ten new species of legionella. *Int J Syst Bact* **35**, 50-59.

Brown, S.L., Bibb, W.F. and McKinney, R.M. (1984). Panvalent antiserum for detection of Legionellae in lung specimens by indirect fluorescent-antibody testing. In *Legionella: Proceedings of the 2nd International Symposium: Washington DC.*, pp. 22-4. Edited by Thornsberry, C., Balows, A., Feeley, J.C. and Jakubowski, W. American Society for Microbiology, Washington.

Brown, A., Lema, M., Ciesielski, M. and Blaser, J. (1985). Combined plasmid and peptide analysis of clinical and environmental *Legionella pneumophila* strains associated with a small cluster of Legionnaires' disease cases. *Infection* **13**, 163-6.

Brown, A., Vickers, R.M., Elder, E.M. *et al.* (1982). Plasmid and surface antigen markers of endemic and epidemic *Legionella pneumophila* strains. *J Clin Microbiol* **16**, 230-35.

Bullen, J.J. (1985). Iron and infection (Editorial). *Eur J Clin Microbiol* **4**, 537-9.

Chandler, F.W., McDade, J.E., Hicklin, M.D. *et al.* (1979). Pathologic findings in guinea-pigs inoculated intraperitoneally with Legionnaires' disease bacterium. *Ann Intern Med* **90**, 671-5.

Chandler, F.W., Roth, K., Callaway, C.S. *et al.* (1980a). Flagella on Legionnaires' disease bacteria: ultrastructural observations. *Ann Intern Med* **93**, 711-14.

Chandler, F.W., Thomason, B.M. and Hébert, G.A. (1980b). Flagella on Legionnaires' disease bacteria in the human lung. *Ann Intern Med* **93**, 715-16.

Chen, G.C.C., Lema, M. and Brown, A. (1984). Plasmid transfer into members of the family Legionellaceae. *J Infect Dis* **150**, 513-16.

Cherry, W.B., Gorman, G.W., Orrison, L.H. *et al.* (1982). *Legionella jordanis*: a new species of *Legionella* isolated from water and sewage. *J Clin Microbiol* **15**, 290-97.

Cherry, W.B., Pittman, B., Harris, P.P. *et al.* (1978). Detection of Legionnaires' disease by direct immunofluorescent staining. *J Clin Microbiol* **8**, 329-38.

Chester, B., Poulos, E.G., Demaray, M.J. *et al.* (1983). Isolation of *Legionella pneumophila* serogroup 1 from blood with nonsupplemented blood cultures bottles. *J Clin Microbiol* **17**, 195-7.

Colbourne, J.S. and Ashworth, J. (1986). Rubbers, water and legionella. *Lancet* **2**, 583.

Colbourne, J.S., Smith, M.G., Fisher-Hoch, S.P. *et al.* (1984). Source of *Legionella pneumophila* infection in a hospital hot water system: materials used in water fittings capable of supporting *L. pneumophila* growth. In *Legionella: Proceedings of the 2nd International Symposium: Washington, D.C.*, pp. 305-7. Edited by Thornsberry, C., Balows, A., Feeley, J.C. and Jakubowski, W. American Society for Microbiology, Washington.

Collins, M.D. and Gilbart, J. (1983). New members of the co-enzyme Q series from the *Legionellaceae*. *FEMS Microbiol Lett* **16**, 251–5.

Conlan, J.W., Baskerville, A. and Ashworth, L.A.E. (1986). Separation of *Legionella pneumophila* proteases and purification of a protease which produces lesions like those of Legionnaires' disease in guinea pig lung. *J Gen Microbiol* **132**, 1565–74

Dennis, P.J., Taylor, J.A. and Barrow, G.I. (1981). Phosphate-buffered low sodium chloride blood agar medium for *Legionella pneumophila*. *Lancet* **2**, 636.

Dennis, P.J., Taylor, J.A., Fitzgeorge, R.B. *et al.* (1982). *Legionella pneumophila* in water plumbing systems. *Lancet* **1**, 949–51.

Dumoff, M. (1979). Direct *in-vitro* isolation of the Legionnaires' disease bacterium in two fatal cases. *Ann Intern Med* **90**, 694–6.

Edelstein, P.H. (1981). Improved semi-selective medium for isolation of *Legionella pneumophila* from contaminated clinical and environmental specimens. *J Clin Microbiol* **14**, 298–303.

Edelstein, P.H., Beer, K.B., Sturge, J.C. *et al.* (1985). Clinical utility of a monoclonal direct fluorescent reagent specific for *Legionella pneumophila*: comparative study with other reagents. *J Clin Microbiol* **22**, 419–21.

Edelstein, P.H., Meyer, R.D. and Finegold, S.M. (1979). Isolation of *Legionella pneumophila* from blood. *Lancet* **1**, 750–1.

Edelstein, P.H., Nakahama, C., Tobin, J.O. *et al.* (1986). Paleoepidemiologic investigation of Legionnaires' disease at Wadsworth Veterans Administration Hospital by using three typing methods for comparison of legionellae from clinical and environmental sources. *J Clin Microbiol*, **23**, 1121–6.

Edwards, R. and Feltham, R.K.A. (1983). Taxonomic implications of the cellular fatty acid content of the Legionellaceae and possibly related species. *FEMS Microbiol Lett* **17**, 251–5.

Faine, S. (1965). Silver staining of spirochaetes in single tissue sections. *J Clin Pathol* **18**, 381–2.

Feeley, J.C., Gibson, R.J., Gorman, G.W. *et al.* (1979). Charcoal yeast extract agar: primary isolation medium for *Legionella pneumophila*. *J Clin Microbiol* **10**, 437–41.

Feeley, J.C., Gorman, G.W., Weaver, R.E. *et al.* (1978). Primary isolation media for Legionnaires' disease bacterium. *J Clin Microbiol* **8**, 320–25.

Fields, B.S., Shotts, E.B., Feeley, J.C. *et al.* (1984). Proliferation of *Legionella pneumophila* as an intracellular parasite of the ciliated protozoan *Tetrahymena pyriformis*. *Appl Environm Microbiol* **47**, 467–71.

Finnerty, W.R., Makula, R.A. and Feeley, J.C. (1979). Cellular lipids of Legionnaires' disease bacterium. *Ann Intern Med* **90**, 631–4.

George, J.R., Pine, L., Reeves, M.W. and Harrell, W.K. (1980). Amino acid requirements of *Legionella pneumophila*. *J. Clin Microbiol* **11**, 286–91.

Gilbart, J. and Collins, M.D. (1985). High-performance liquid chromatographic analysis of ubiquinones from new *Legionella* species. *FEMS Microbiol Lett* **26**, 77–82.

Glick, T.H., Gregg, M.B., Berman, B. *et al.* (1978). An epidemic of unknown aetiology in a Health Department. *Am J Epidemiol* **167**, 149–60.

Gorman, G.W., Feeley, J.C., Steigerwalt, A. *et al.* (1985). *Legionella anisa*: a new species of *Legionella* isolated from potable waters and a cooling tower. *Appl Environm Microbiol* **49**, 305–9.

Gosting, L.H., Cabrian, K., Sturge, J.C. and Goldstein, L.C. (1984). Identification of a species-specific antigen in *Legionella pneumophila* by a monoclonal antibody. *J Clin Microbiol* **20**, 1031–5.

Greaves, P.W. (1980). New methods for the isolation of *Legionella pneumophila*. *J Clin Pathol* **33**, 581–4.

Grimont, P.A.D., Grimont, F., Desplaces, N. and Tchen, P. (1985). DNA probe specific for *Legionella pneumophila*. *J Clin Microbiol* **21**, 431–7.

Groothuis, D.G., Veenendaal, H.R., Meenhorst, P.L. (1984). Serogrouping of Legionellae by slide agglutination test with monospecific sera. In *Legionella: Proceedings of the 2nd International Symposium: Washington, DC.*, pp. 35–7. Edited by Thornsberry, C., Balows, A., Feeley, J.C. and Jakubowski, W. American Society for Microbiology, Washington.

Guerrant, G.O., Lambert, M.S. and Moss, C.W. (1979). Identification of diaminopimelic acid in the Legionnaires' disease bacterium. *J Clin Microbiol* **10**, 815–18.

Hébert, G.A., Callaway, C.S. and Ewing, E.P. Jr. (1984). Comparison of *Legionella pneumophila*, *L. micdadei*, *L. bozemanii* and *L. dumoffii* by transmission electron microscopy. *J Clin Microbiol* **19**, 116–21.

Hébert, G.A., Steigerwalt, A.G. and Brenner, D.J. (1980). *Legionella micdadei* species nova: classification of a third species of *Legionella* associated with human pneumonia. *Curr Microbiol* **3**, 255–7.

Hindahl, M.S. and Iglewski, B.H. (1984). Isolation and characterization of the *Legionella pneumophila* outer membrane. *J Bact* **159**, 107–13.

Hoffman, P. (1984). Bacterial physiology. In *Legionella: Proceedings of the 2nd International Symposium: Washingon, DC.*, pp 61–7. Edited by Thornsberry, C., Balows, A., Feeley, J., Jakubowski, W. American Society for Microbiology, Washington.

Holden, E.P., Winkler, H.H., Wood, D.O. and Leinbach, E.D. (1984). Intracellular growth of *Legionella pneumophila* within Acanthamoeba castellani Neff. *Infect Immun* **45**, 18–24.

Holmes, R.L. (1982). Aniline blue-containing buffered charcoal yeast extract medium for presumptive identification of legionella species. *J Clin Microbiol* **15**, 723–4.

Horwitz, M.A. (1984). Interactions between *Legionella pneumophila* and human mononuclear phagocytes. In *Legionella: Proceedings of the 2nd International Symposium: Washington, DC.*, pp. 159–66. Edited by Thornsberry, C., Balows, A., Feeley, J.C. and Jakubowski, W. American Society for Microbiology, Washington.

Johnson, S.R., Schalla, W.O., Wong, K.H. and Perkins, G.H. (1982). Simple transparent medium for study of *Legionellae*. *J Clin Microbiol* **15**, 342–4.

Joly, J.R., McKinney, R.M., Tobin, J.O. *et al.* (1986). Development of a standardized subgrouping scheme for *Legionella pneumophila* serogroup 1 using monoclonal antibodies. *J Clin Microbiol* **23**, 768–71.

Joly, J.R. and Winn, W.C. (1984). Correlation of subtypes of *Legionella pneumophila* defined by monoclonal antibodies with epidemiological classfication of cases and environmental sources. *J Infect Dis* **150**, 667–71.

Karr, D.E., Bibb, W.F. and Moss, C.W. (1982). Isoprenoid quinones of the genus *Legionella*. *J Clin Microbiol* **15**, 1044–8.

Kaufmann, A.F., McDade, J.E., Patton, C.M. *et al.* (1981). Pontiac fever: Isolation of the etiologic agent (*Legionella pneumophila*) and demonstration of its mode of transmission. *Am J Epidemiol* **114**, 337–47.

Keathley, J.D. and Winn, W.C. (1984). Comparison of media for recovery of Legionella pneumophila clinical isolates. In *Legionella: Proceedings of the 2nd International Symposium: Washington, DC.*, pp. 19–20. Edited by Thornsberry, C., Balows, A., Feeley, J.C. and Jakubowski, W. American Society for Microbiology, Washington.

Ketel, R.J. van, Schegget, J. ter, Zanen, H.C. (1984). Molecular epidemiology of *Legionella pneumophila* serogroup 1. *J Clin Microbiol* **20**, 362–4.

Kohler, R.B., Allen, S.D. and Wilson, E.R. (1984). Cross-reacting antigens in a radiometric assay for urinary *Legionella pneumophila* antigen. In *Legionella: Proceedings of the 2nd International Symposium: Washington, DC.*, pp. 40–42. Edited by Thornsberry, C., Balows, A., Feeley, J.C. and Jakubowski, W. American Society for Microbiology, Washington.

McDade, J.E., Brenner, D.J. and Bozeman, M. (1979). Legionnaires' disease bacterium isolated in 1947. *Ann Intern Med* **90**, 659–61.

McDade, J.E., Shepperd, C.C. and Fraser, D.W. *et al*. (1977). Legionnaires' disease. Isolation of a bacterium and demonstration of its role in other respiratory disease. *N Engl J Med* **297**, 1197–1203.

Macrae, A.D., Appleton, P.N., Laverick, A. (1979). Legionnaires' disease in Nottingham, England. *Ann Intern Med* **90**, 580–83.

Martin, R.S., Marrie, T.J., Best, L. *et al*. (1984). Isolation of *Legionella pneumophila* from the blood of a patient with Legionnaires' disease. *Can Med Ass J* **131**, 1085–7.

Mather, W.E., Plouffe, J.F. and Para, M.F. (1983). Plasmid profiles of clinical and environmental isolates of *Legionella pneumophila* serogroup 1. *J Clin Microbiol* **18**, 1422–3.

Moss, C.W., Karr, D.E. and Dees, S.B. (1981). Cellular fatty acid composition of *Legionella longbeachae* sp. nov. *J Clin Microbiol* **14**, 692–4.

Müller, H.E. (1984). Proteoloytic action in actively growing Legionellae. In *Legionella: Proceedings of the 2nd International Symposium: Washington, DC.*, pp. 85–6. Edited by Thornsberry, C., Balows, A., Feeley, J.C. and Jakubowski, W. American Society for Microbiology, Washington.

Niedeveld, C.J., Pet, F.M. and Meenhorst, P.L. (1986). Effect of rubbers and their constituents on proliferation of *Legionella pneumophila* in naturally contaminated hot water. *Lancet* **2**, 180–84.

Nolte, F.S., Hollick, G.E. and Robertson, R.G. (1982). Enzymatic activities of *Legionella pneumophila* and *Legionella*-like organisms. *J Clin Microbiol* **15**, 175–7.

Quinn, F.D. and Weinberg, E.D. (1984). Susceptibility of *Legionella pneumophila* to iron-binding agents. In *Legionella: Proceedings of the 2nd International Symposium: Washington, DC.*, pp. 77–9. Edited by Thornsberry, C., Balows, A., Feeley, J.C. and Jakubowski, W. American Society for Microbiology, Washington.

Report. (1981). Bacterial nomenclature. *Wkly Epidem Rec* **56**, 399.

Rihs, J.D., Yu, V.L., Zuravleff, J.J. *et al*. (1985). Isolation of *Legionella pneumophila* from blood with the BACTEC system: a prospective study yielding positive results. *J Clin Microbiol* **22**, 422–4.

Rodgers, F.G. (1979). Ultrastructure of *Legionella pneumophila*. *J Clin Pathol* **32**, 1195–1202.

Rodgers, F.G. and Davey, M.R. (1982). Ultrastructure of the cell envelope layers and surface details of *Legionella pneumophila*. *J Gen Microbiol* **128**, 1547–57.

Rodgers, F.G., Greaves, P.W., Macrae, A.D. and Lewis, M.J. (1980). Electron microscopic evidence of flagella and pili on *Legionella pneumophila*. *J. Clin Pathol* **33**, 1184–8.

Rodgers, F.G. and Macrae, A.D. (1979). Immunoferritin electron microscopy in legionellosis. *Lancet* **1**, 786.

Rodgers, F.G. and Oldham, L.J. (1984). Intracellular and extracellular replication of *Legionella pneumophila* in cells *in vitro*. In *Legionella: Proceedings of the 2nd International Symposium: Washington, DC.*, pp. 184–6. Edited by Thornsberry, C., Balows, A., Feeley, J.C. and Jakubowski, W. American Society for Microbiology, Washington.

Rowbotham, T.J. (1980). Preliminary report on the pathogenicity of *Legionella pneumophila* for fresh water and soil amoeba. *J Clin Pathol* **33**, 1179–83.

Rowbotham, T.J. (1984). Legionellae and amoeba. In *Legionella: Proceedings of the 2nd International Symposium: Washington, DC.*, pp. 325–7. Edited by Thornsberry, C., Balows, A., Feeley, J.C. and Jakubowski, W. American Society for Microbiology, Washington.

Schofield, G.M. and Locci, R. (1985a). The persistence of *Legionella pneumophila* in non-sterile, sterile and artificial hard waters and their growth pattern on tap washer fittings. *J Appl Bacteriol* **59**, 519–27.

Schofield, G.M. and Locci, R. (1985b). Colonization of components of a model hot water system by *Legionella pneumophila*. *J. Appl Bact* **58**, 151–62.

Schofield, G.M. and Wright, A.E. (1984). Survival of *Legionella pneumophila* in a model hot water distribution system. *J Gen Microbiol* **130**, 1751–6.

Tenover, F.C., Carlson, L., Goldstein, L. *et al.* (1985). Confirmation of *Legionella pneumophila* cultures with a fluorescein-labelled monoclonal antibody. *J Clin Microbiol* **21**, 983–4.

Thacker, W.L., Benson, R.F., Wilkinson, H.W. *et al.* (1986). 11th serogroup of *Legionella pneumophila* isolated from a patient with fatal pneumonia. *J Clin Microbiol* **23**, 1146–7.

Thacker, W.L., Plikaytis, B.B. and Wilkinson, H.W. (1985a). Identification of *Legionella* species and 33 serogroups with the slide agglutination test. *J Clin Microbiol* **21**, 779–82.

Thacker, W.L., Wilkinson, H.W., Plikaytis, B.B. *et al.* (1985b). Second serogroup of *Legionella feeleii* strains isolated from humans. *J Clin Microbiol* **22**, 1–4.

Thomason, B.M., Chandler, F.W. and Hollis, D.G. (1979). Flagella on Legionnaires' disease bacteria: an interim report. *Ann Intern Med* **91**, 224–6.

Thorpe, T.C. and Miller, R.D. (1984). Characterization of an extracellular haemolysin from *Legionella pneumophila*. In *Legionella: Proceedings of the 2nd International Symposium: Washington, DC.*, pp. 97–8. Edited by Thornsberry, C., Balows, A., Feeley, J.C. and Jakubowski, W. American Society for Microbiology, Washington.

Tison, D.L., Pope, D.H., Cherry, W.B. and Fliermans, C.B. (1980). Growth on *Legionella pneumophila* in association with blue-green algae (cyanobacteria). *Appl Environm Microbiol* **39**, 456–9.

Vickers, R.M., Brown, A. and Garrity, G.M. (1981). Dye-containing buffered charcoal yeast extract medium for differentiation of members of the family *Legionellaceae*. *J Clin Microbiol* **13**, 380–82.

Vickers, R.M. and Yu, V.L. (1984). Clinical and laboratory differentiation of *Legionellaceae* family members with pigment production and fluorescence on media supplemented with aromatic substrates. *J Clin Microbiol* **19**, 583–7.

Wadowsky, R.M. and Yee, R.B. (1981). Glycine-containing selective medium for isolation of *Legionellaceae* from environmental specimens. *Appl Environm Microbiol* **42**, 768–72.

Wadowsky, R.M. and Yee, R.B. (1983). Satellite growth of *Legionella pneumophila* with an environmental isolate of *Flavobacterium breve*. *Appl Environm Microbiol* **46**, 1447–9.

Watkins, I.D., Tobin, J.O.H., Dennis, P.J. *et al.* (1985). *Legionella pneumophila* serogroup 1 subgrouping by monoclonal antibodies – an epidemiological tool. *J Hyg Camb* **95**, 211–16.

Wilkinson, H.W. and Fikes, B.J. (1981). Detection of cell-associated or soluble antigens of *Legionella pneumophila* serogroups 1 to 6, *Legionella bozemanii*, *Legionella dumoffii*, *Legionella gormanii*, and *Legionella micdadei* by staphylococcal coagglutination tests. *J Clin Microbiol* **14**, 322–5.

Winn, W.C. and Myerowitz, R.L. (1981). The pathology of Legionella pneumonias. *Human Pathology* **12**, 401–22.

Wong, K.H. and Feeley, J.C. (1983). Antigens and toxic components of Legionella in pathogenesis and immunity. *Zbl Bakt I Abt Orig A* **255**, 133–8.

Wong, M.C., Ewing, E.P., Callaway, C.S. and Peacock, W.L. (1980). Intracellular multiplication of *Legionella pneumophila* in cultured human embryonic lung fibroblasts. *Infect Immun* **28**, 1014–18.

2 Legionella Species

Terminology and classification

The categorization of organisms is important even if the procedures involved may on occasion seem formidable. Taxonomy, embodying the principles of classification, has to be focused on the properties of a bacterial genus or species. For the Legionellaceae, definition as a genus has drawn on characteristics which include morphology and ultrastructure, staining reactions, chemical including cellular fatty acid composition, growth capability, biochemical reactions, enzymatic profiles and isoprenoid quinone content, antigenic patterns, DNA genome size and guanine plus cytosine ratios, plus genetic homology. Newly identified organisms must also be compared with known species to ensure they are distinct.

When first classified as *Legionella pneumophila*, genus novum, species nova (Brenner *et al.*, 1979) the newly established genus had only one species. Since that time further bacteria with similar though not always identical properties have been recovered from ill patients and from a variety of environmental sources. Designation of a gradually increasing number of species has followed, together with discussion on the desirability or otherwise of creating new genera. At present this last matter is in abeyance. Within the *L. pneumophila* species, antigenic differences among certain newly isolated strains had led to subdivision of these into a number of serogroups (McKinney *et al.*, 1979) based on specific immunofluorescence of intact organisms. The extraction and purification of soluble group-specific lipopolysaccharide antigens as well as shared protein antigens has supported this (Wong *et al.*, 1979; Pearlman *et al.*, 1985).

Legionella pneumophila

The serogroups of *L. pneumophila* which have been classified are listed in Table 2.1. Others will be added as and when identified. The initial observation of antigenic distinctiveness among *L. pneumophila* strains came from the finding that a bacterium from lung tissue of a patient with pneumonia in Togus, Maine, USA, which had the other features of a legionella organism, did not fluoresce with Knoxville, a broadly reacting (SG1) antiserum conjugate, yet fluoresced strongly with its homologous antiserum conjugate.

Table 2.1 *Legionella pneumophila* serogroups

Serogroup	Type strain	Other representative strains[xx]
1	Philadelphia 1	Knoxville 1, *Pontiac* 1, Flint 1, *Olda*, *Bellingham* 1, etc
2	Togus 1	Atlanta 1, 2, 4, Macon 1
3	Bloomington 2[x]	Burlington 4, Detroit 5
4	Los Angeles 1	Baltimore 2
5	Dallas 1[x]	Dallas 2[x], 3[x], Burlington 1[x], Cambridge 2
6	Chicago 2	Chicago 3, 4, Houston, 2, Oxford, Bethesda 1
7	Chicago 8[x]	Dallas 5
8	Concord 3	
9	IN-23-GI-C2 (Leiden)[x]	Wadsworth 83–100A " 83–103A
10	Leiden 1	Other Leiden isolates
11	797-PA-H	

[x] Environmental isolates
[xx] Serogroup 1 strains underlined represent major subgroups (see Watkins *et al.*, 1985)

Almost simultaneously two further isolates, Bloomington 2 and Los Angeles 1, were shown to be distinct not only from Knoxville and Togus 1 but also from each other. From this, recognition of the first four serogroups evolved (McKinney *et al.*, 1979; Wilkinson *et al.*, 1979). The Bloomington 2 (SG3) strain was an environmental isolate recovered from creek water during studies of a *L. pneumophila* (SG1) outbreak at Bloomington, Indiana (Morris *et al.*, 1979). It was established after isolation of a strain from lung tissue of an immunosuppressed patient dying from pneumonia that this serogroup could also be a human pathogen (Watts *et al.*, 1980). The Los Angeles (SG4) strain was recovered initially from lung tissue of a pneumonic patient under treatment with corticosteroids (Edelstein *et al.*, 1978).

A fifth serogroup, represented by Dallas 1 as type strain, was recovered from cooling tower water during investigations of a *L. pneumophila* (SG1) outbreak at a convention in Dallas, Texas (England *et al.*, 1980). About the same time, however, a strain belonging to this serogroup and isolated from lung tissue, had caused a fatal pneumonia in a patient on prednisolone for chronic lymphatic leukaemia in Cambridge, England (Nagington *et al.*, 1979).

A sixth serogroup of which Chicago 2 is the type strain was first identified in lung tissue from three renal transplant patients with pneumonia in Chicago, Illinois (McKinney *et al.*, 1980). Similar strains were recovered from two renal transplant patients with pneumonia in Oxford, England (Tobin *et al.*, 1980). Though found cross-reactive with serogroup 3 the presence of a distinct as well as shared antigens supported its placement in a separate serogroup (Taylor and Harrison, 1979).

The seventh serogroup was established from two strains with similar serological characteristics though distinct from serogroups 1–6 (Bibb *et al.*, 1983). One strain, an environmental isolate obtained in a survey of private residences in Chicago was named Chicago 8 and became the type strain. The other strain, Dallas 5 from Texas came from post-mortem lung of a patient with pneumonia.

An eighth serogroup was established with Concord 3, as the new strain. This isolate was recovered from post-mortem lung of a patient with pneumonia in California (Bissett *et al.*, 1983). In immunofluorescence tests some cross-reaction with serogroups 4 and 5 was observed though the response to the homologous antibody was considerably greater. By reciprocal immuno-electrophoresis tests with absorbed and unabsorbed sera against Concord 3 and Dallas 1 (SG5) antigens it appeared that the cross-reacting components could be absorbed out leaving distinct and unshared major antigens. This was sufficient to warrant a new serogroup.

The ninth serogroup has been based on four closely related strains. Two were recovered from immunocompetent patients who had pneumonia, one from post-mortem lung tissue of a fatal case from Abingdon, Virginia and the other from a lung biopsy of a surviving patient who came from Loma Linda, California. Two strains were environmental isolates, one was from water samples collected in Leiden University Hospital, Holland, the other, a previously unidentified *L. pneumophila* strain, was isolated from shower water in South Africa (Edelstein *et al.*, 1984). Apart from minor cross-reactions with strains from serogroups 1, 3 and 5 which could be absorbed out, the new serogroup remained distinct serologically. Its type strain is IN-23-G1-C2 from Leiden.

The tenth serogroup, of which Leiden 1 is the designated type strain, had been a cause of nosocomial legionella infections among immunocompromised patients in Leiden University Hospital, Holland (Meenhorst *et al.*, 1985). Strains were recovered both from affected patients and from the hospital's potable or drinkable water supply. Although cross-reactions occurred with serogroups 4, 5 and 8 absorption tests removed antigens in common while leaving the specific and distinct major antigen of the new serogroup.

The eleventh serogroup, of which 797-PA-H is the designated type strain, was recovered from endotracheal aspirate and also lung tissue from a patient with fatal pneumonia in Pittsburgh, Pennsylvania. It had the characteristics of *Legionella pneumophila* but did not cross-react with the other serogroups. It did cross-react, but only minimally, with the Lansing 3 strain, an as yet unclassified legionella-like species (Thacker *et al.*, 1986).

It remains a feature of the *L. pneumophila* species that, given the opportunity, all can act as human pathogens, regardless of serogroup, with pneumonia the common and most frequent illness. Serogroup 1 organisms have, however, been the major aetiological agents recovered from outbreaks and sporadic infections in previously healthy as well as immunosuppressed persons (Wilkinson *et al.*, 1983). This may be the result of a wider environmental distribution (Fliermans *et al.*, 1981), a greater possession of virulence factors among such strains or a combination of both circumstances. With other serogroups the illness occurs more noticeably in disadvantaged patients.

This expanding range of serogroups has entailed a need to include multiple antigens in serological screening tests for suspected legionellosis. Further, the antibody reactions of patients to infection can be both variable and confusing. Some show a monospecific serogroup response of clear diagnostic import, others present broader intergroup effects which may develop at different stages of the illness and vary in extent and duration. Due to this clouding of serological responses, attempted recovery of the causative agent from patient material has become an increasingly important objective. These variable effects stem from the antigenic content of legionella organisms. In addition to the specific heat-stable serogroup surface antigen, electrophoresis tests have detected as many as 30 protein antigens among *L. pneumophila* strains (Joly and Kenny, 1982; Pearlman *et al.*, 1985). A smaller number of these common antigens were shared with other legionella species. It has also emerged from studies of electrophoretic mobilities of enzymes encoded by structural genes that polymorphism among strains is considerable (Selander *et al.*, 1985). There is further evidence that flagellar antigen from the different species is closely related (Brenner *et al.*, 1985; Elliott and Johnson, 1981; Rodgers and Laverick, 1984). Whether this may be of diagnostic value or have any effect on the course of the disease is at present uncertain.

As well as the cross-reactions observed between serogroups, strain differences within groups are becoming evident. In early immuno-fluorescence studies at the Centres for Disease Control, Atlanta (McKinney *et al.*, 1979), considerable variations in titre between *L. pneumophila* serogroup 1 strains were recorded (Table 2.2). Other studies, with human lung extracts as antigen reacting with guinea-pig antisera similarly provided evidence of a difference in homologous and heterologous responses (Macrae *et al.*, 1979). Strains became separable into subgroups with selectively absorbed sera (Brown *et al.*, 1982; Thomason and Bibb, 1984) and then with monoclonal antibodies (Joly *et al.*, 1983, 1986; Watkins and Tobin, 1984; Watkins *et al.*, 1985), a technique which can provide bacterial markers, of use in epidemiological investigations. Whether the observed variations in virulence or association with disease (Bollin *et al.*, 1985) are static or can be altered is not however clear. Besides serogroup 1, diversity among sero-group 5 isolates has been reported (Garrity *et al.*, 1982; Watkins and Tobin 1984).

Problems with culture had made identification of legionella strains from both human and environmental sources dependent on serology, mainly by the use of immunofluorescence techniques. A possible difficulty lay in the

Table 2.2 *Legionella pneumophila* serogroup 1 strains

| | *Fluorescent antibody titres* [*] | |
| | Antibody | Conjugate |
Strain	Knoxville 1	Togus 1
Knoxville 1	1024	< 16
Philadelphia 3	4096	< 16
Pontiac 1	2048	< 16
Detroit 1	16	< 16
Olda	16	< 16
Bellingham 1	16	< 16

[*] Abstracted from Table 1 in McKinney *et al.*, 1979

fact that cross-reactions might be found between legionella species and other, particularly Gram-negative organisms. Some strains of *Pseudomonas fluorescens* and *alcaligenes, Bacteroides fragilis* and the *Flavobacterium-Xanthomonas* group were found to cross-react in varying degree though not consistently. This effect needs to be borne in mind when interpreting results (Edelstein *et al.*, 1980; Orrison *et al.*, 1983).

Reports of a serological overlap with other respiratory pathogens such as *Mycoplasma pneumoniae* or *Chlamydia psittaci* have not been confirmed either in Britain (Taylor *et al.*, 1980) or in the United States (Wentworth and Stiefel, 1982; Edelstein, 1984). In some instances an apparent overlap could follow a dual infection or be an anamnestic response from a past illness.

Other legionella species

Named legionella species which are distinct from *Legionella pneumophila* are shown in Table 2.3. Others are in the process of classification. Isolated both from patients, often with pneumonia, and from aqueous environments they were at first called atypical legionella-like organisms (ALLO) though this nomenclature was abandoned when it became apparent there were legionella species other than *L. pneumophila*. Definition of their characteristics including a lack of relatedness to established species has resulted in steady expansion of numbers in the group.

L. bozemanii serogroup 1
The Wiga type strain of this serogroup had been recovered in 1959 by guinea-pig and egg inoculation from the lung of a patient dying of pneumonia after attending a course on the use of underwater breathing apparatus (Bozeman *et al.*, 1968). It remained unclassified for over 20 years except that though morphologically similar, it differed from the Tatlock and Olda strains in guinea-pig cross-immunity tests.

A second strain (MI-15) was isolated in 1979 from lung tissue in a fatal infection which followed accidental immersion in a swampy freshwater lake. This strain was cultured directly on CYE agar as well as by guinea-pig and egg inoculation (Cordes *et al.*, 1979).

Both strains were found to possess features associated with the legionella family of organisms and shared some antigens, though not serogroup specific antigen, with *L. pneumophila*. They were closely related to each other, both immunologically and by DNA hybridization, but were otherwise sufficiently distinctive to be named as a separate species (Brenner *et al.*, 1980).

Since then *L. bozemanii* has been associated with further cases of pneumonia in the United States (Sobell *et al.*, 1983) and in Europe (Mitchell *et al.*, 1984).

As the criterion, that within the legionella genus there should be at least 25 per cent of DNA sequence homology was not fulfilled, a new *Fluoribacter* genus with *F. bozemanae* as a member was proposed (Garrity *et al.*, 1980). This proposal was not accepted for inclusion in the latest edition of Bergey's Manual of Determinative Bacteriology (Brenner *et al.*, 1982). Reasons for not applying it have been elaborated (Brenner *et al.*, 1985).

Table 2.3 Other legionella species

Species		Type strain	Other strains	Synonym
Legionella bozemanii	serogroup 1	Wiga	MI-12, (GA-PH)	*Fluoribacter bozemanae*
"	serogroup 2	Toronto 3		
Legionella dumoffii		NY-23	Tex-KL	*Fluoribacter dumoffii*
Legionella micdadei		Tatlock	Heba, Pittsburgh Pneumonia Agent (PPA)	*Tatlockia micdadei*
Legionella gormanii	serogroup 1	LS-13	Other environmental isolates	*Fluoribacter gormanii*
Legionella longbeachae	serogroup 1	LB 4	LA24, Concord 1, Atlanta 5	
"	serogroup 2	Tucker 1	ABB9	
Legionella jordanis		BL-540		
Legionella oakridgensis		OR-10	Other OR strains	
Legionella wadsworthii		Wadsworth 81–716A		
Legionella feeleii	serogroup 1	WO-44C-C3	425-MI-H, 713-MI-E	
"	serogroup 2	691-WI-H	693-WI-H	
Legionella sainthelensi		Mt. St. Helens 4	Other Mt. St. Helens strains	
Legionella anisa		WA-316-C3	Other environmental isolates	
Legionella maceachernii		PX-1-G2-E2	SC-73-C2	
Legionella jamestowniensis		JA-26-GI-E2		
Legionella rubrilucens		WA-270A-C2		
Legionella erytha		SE-32A-C8		
Legionella spiritensis		Mt. St. Helens 9		
Legionella hackeliae	serogroup 1	Lansing 2		
"	serogroup 2	798-PA-H		
Legionella parisiensis		PF-209C-C2		
Legionella cherrii		ORW	ORB ORZ, SC-65-C3	
Legionella steigerwaltii		SC-18-C9		
Legionella santicrucis		SC-63-C7		
Legionella israelensis		Bercovier 4	Bercovier 5, 7	

L. bozemanii **serogroup 2**

The Toronto 3 type strain of this serogroup came from lung aspirate of a patient with pneumonia indistinguishable from other legionella pneumonias. The strain showed 90 per cent DNA relatedness to the *L. bozemanii* serogroup 1 (Wiga) strain and had a similar fatty acid and ubiquinone content. Serologically it cross-reacted with the Wiga strain and with *L. longbeachae* serogroup 2 but could be distinguished after absorption tests (Tang *et al.*, 1984).

L. dumoffii

The NY 23 type strain came from cooling tower water in New York during investigations of legionellosis outbreaks in that city. It was an environmental isolate not associated with disease. A serologically similar strain, named Tex-KL, was recovered from post-mortem lung of a patient who developed severe pneumonia in Texas. With cultural characteristics of the legionella family and fatty acid profiles similar to the Wiga strain the two strains nevertheless showed minimal DNA relatedness to both *L. bozemanii* and *L. pneumophila* species. They were apportioned to a separate species and named *L. dumoffii* (Brenner *et al.*, 1980). The suggestion that, like *L. bozemanii*, they should form part of a separate genus with the name *Fluoribacter dumoffii* (Garrity *et al.*, 1980) has not been sustained. In a strain isolated from an immuno-suppressed patient with pneumonia, phenotypic variation has been reported. Unlike the type strain it failed to produce browning of tyrosine-containing buffered yeast extract medium (Edelstein and Pryor, 1985).

L. micdadei

The Tatlock type strain was recovered in 1943 by guinea-pig intraperitoneal inoculation with blood from a soldier with 'Fort-Bragg' fever, though the organism appeared unrelated to the illness. In 1959, the HEBA strain was isolated by the same technique from the blood of a patient with suspected pityriasis rosea. In 1979, the Pittsburgh Pneumonia Agent (PPA) was derived from lung tissue of renal transplant patients who had suffered from pneumonia.

These three strains, diverse in source and time, were found to be of the legionella family, antigenically and phenotypically similar, with high DNA relatedness to each other but not to *L. pneumophila*, *L. bozemanii* or *L. dumoffi*. They constituted a distinct species and were named *L. micdadei* Hébert *et al.*, 1980). Again, a proposal that they were a separate genus and should be named *Tatlockia micdadei* (Garrity *et al.*, 1980) has not been sustained.

L. gormanii

The LS-13 strain came from moist soil collected from a creek bank during investigations of a legionella outbreak at a golf club in Atlanta. The organism was distinguishable by specific immunofluorescence from other recognized species of legionella including *L. pneumophila*. Its fatty acid profile was similar to that of *L. bozemanii* and *L. dumoffii*. From DNA homology studies it appeared to be a distinct species and although represented by a single strain was named *L. gormanii* (Morris *et al.*, 1980). The features in common with *L. bozemanii* and *L. dumoffii* led to its inclusion in the proposed genus *Fluoribacter* (Garrity *et al.*, 1980) but this again has not been sustained. Since the original isolate, the species has been recovered infrequently from other environmental sources (Christensen *et al.*, 1984).

L. longbeachae serogroup 1
The Long Beach (LB) 4 type strain of this serogroup was one of four Gramnegative immunologically similar bacteria isolated from tracheal aspirates or lung tissue of patients with severe pneumonia. These organisms had the characteristics of the Legionellaceace and, except for inability to hydrolyse hippurate, resembled *L. pneumophila* culturally and in fatty acid composition but differed serologically. They showed close DNA relatedness to each other but only at a low level to other species and were categorized as a new species (McKinney *et al.*, 1981).

L. longbeachae serogroup 2
The Tucker 1 type strain of this serogroup was isolated from lung tissue of a patient with a fatal pneumonia. The organism had the characteristics of the Legionellaceae and it showed close DNA relatedness to *L. longbeachae* serogroup 1. Though some cross-reaction with serogroup 1 had been observed this could be removed by absorption hence its designation as a distinct serogroup (Bibb *et al.*, 1981). In slide agglutination tests a minor cross-reaction was also noted between serogroup 2 antiserum and *L. jordanis* (Thacker *et al.*, 1983).

L. jordanis
The BL-540 type strain was obtained, as an environmental isolate by guinea-pig and egg inoculation then CYE agar culture, from water from the Jordan river, Bloomington, Indiana. The water was collected during investigation of an outbreak of legionnaires' disease, caused by *L. pneumophila* serogroup 1. A closely related strain ABB-9, also an environmental isolate, came from effluent at a sewage disposal plant in Georgia. These strains were found to be similar both serologically and by DNA relatedness but were distinct from other known legionella species except for a minor cross-reaction with *L. bozemanii*. Their fatty acid profile resembled that of *L. bozemanii* and *L. micdadei* rather than *L. pneumophila*. From these characteristics the new species were designated (Cherry *et al.*, 1982). A strain which caused human infection, was recovered from lung-tissues and then identified as *L. jordanis* (Thacker *et al.*, 1983).

L. oakridgensis
The OR-10 type strain and five other environmental isolates were recovered from cooling tower water from a number of sites in Pennsylvania, with four additional strains from Minnesota. They all showed close immunological and DNA relatedness to each other but differed in these respects from other known legionella species. They are said to be non-motile, lacking flagella but how absolute this is for water-borne organisms is uncertain. Also, unlike other legionella species, except for some strains of *L. jordanis*, they do not require added L-cysteine when subcultured (Orrison *et al.*, 1983).

L. wadsworthii

The Wadsworth 81-716A type strain was isolated from the sputum of an immunocompromised patient with severe pneumonia. It had the characteristics of a legionella species with a branched chain fatty acid content essentially similar to *L. jordanis* or *L. bozemanii* but differing from *L. pneumophila* or *L. micdadei*. It was distinct from other legionella species immunologically and in its DNA relatedness and was designated a new species (Edelstein *et al.*, 1982).

L. feeleii serogroup 1

The WO-44C type strain was isolated from a sample of a coolant mixture of water (at least 88 per cent) and oil. This was used in an engine assembly plant in Windsor, Ontario, in which there had been a sudden, self-limited outbreak of Pontiac fever, ascribed to contaminated aerosol spray. The strain showed many of the features of a legionella organism. It required L-cysteine for growth and could, like *L. pneumophila*, hydrolyse hippurate but did not produce gelatinase. It contained branched-chain fatty acids similar to other legionella species but was distinct from them antigenically and by DNA relatedness sufficiently to be designated a new species (Herwaldt *et al.*, 1984). An identical serogroup 1 strain has also been isolated from the sputum of a patient with pneumonia (Thacker *et al.*, 1983).

L. feeleii serogroup 2

The type strain, 691-WI-H, one of three strains from patients with pneumonia together with a further environmental isolate were all allocated to the *L. feeleii* species on the basis of their DNA relationship. Serologically distinct from serogroup 1 they were accorded separate status as serogroup 2 (Thacker *et al.*, 1985).

L. sainthelensi

The Mt. St. Helens 4 type strain, one of six similar strains, was recovered together with several other legionella species, from water samples during 1981 investigations in the area by Mt. St. Helens, Washington, scene of a devastating volcanic eruption in 1980. Possessing the characteristics of Legionellaceae the strain differs by DNA relatedness and antigenicity from other species, although it has given some cross-reactions with both *L. longbeachae* serogroups and with *L. oakridgensis* (Campbell *et al.*, 1984).

Information on the characterization of a further 12' species, 11 being environmental isolates is now available (Bercovier *et al.*, 1986; Brenner *et al.*, 1985; Gorman *et al.*, 1985; Wilkinson *et al.*, 1985a) and has been abstracted. The studies of their phenotypic traits are continuing.

L. anisa

The WA-316-C3 type strain, from a water sample taken at a Los Angeles hospital in 1981, was one of four similar hospital-based strains from Los Angeles and Chicago. A fifth strain was recovered from cooling tower water in Jamestown, New York. All possessed the biochemical and other properties of Legionellaceae though none was directly associated with human disease.

They showed cross-reactions with *L. bozemanii* serogroup 2 and with *L. longbeachae* serogroup 2 in fluorescent antibody tests and a relation to *L. parisiensis* in DNA studies but were sufficiently distinctive to be classed as a new species.

L. maceachernii
The PX-1-G2-E2 type strain came from water from a home evaporator-cooler in Phoenix, Arizona in 1979, and was isolated initially by guinea-pig and egg yolk sac inoculation. A further strain, also an environmental isolate but cultured directly on CYE agar, came from St. Thomas, Virgin Islands in 1982. The two strains were identical from their DNA relatedness. Characteristically legionellas, they were distinct from other species apart from some cross-reaction with *L. micdadei*. They showed no autofluorescence and did not produce beta-lactamase. This species has since been recovered from lung of an immunocompromised patient with fatal pneumonia (Wilkinson *et al.*, 1985b).

L. jamestowniensis
The JA-26-G1-E2 type strain came from wet soil at Jamestown, New York in the course of investigation of a legionella outbreak. It was recovered in late 1979 by guinea-pig and egg yolk sac inoculation followed by transfer to CYE agar. It was not associated with human illness. It was found to be a legionella but did not autofluoresce and was a distinct species with low relatedness to the other species.

L. rubrilucens
The WA-270A-C2 type strain was recovered from tap water in Los Angeles, California in 1980. It autofluoresces red and although oxidase negative its other reactions are typical of legionella. It shows considerable DNA relatedness to *L. erythra* and to a less extent to the non-fluorescing *L. spiritensis*.

L. erythra
The SE-32A-C8 type strain came from cooling tower water from Seattle, Washington in 1981. It autofluoresces red, is oxidase positive and forms a distinct species. It shows most DNA relatedness to *L. rubrilucens* but again also to some extent to *L. spiritensis*.

L. spiritensis
The Mt. St. Helens 9 type strain was recovered from water from Spirit Lake, in the vicinity of Mt. St. Helens, Washington in 1981. Like *L. pneumophila* it may hydrolyse hippurate and is oxidase positive. Though it does not autofluoresce or cross-react by specific immunofluorescence with other species it shows considerable DNA relatedness to the red autofluorescing species, in particular *L. rubrilucens*.

L. hackeliae serogroup 1
The Lansing 2 type strain was isolated from a bronchial biopsy specimen from a female patient with pneumonia at Ann Arbor, Michigan in 1981. It was weakly oxidase positive and does not autofluoresce, nor cross-react with

other species but does minimally with *L. hackeliae* serogroup 2 with which it also shows high DNA relatedness.

L. hackeliae serogroup 2
The 798-PA-H type strain came from a percutaneous lung aspirate from an immunocompromised female patient with pneumonia at Pittsburgh, Pennsylvania. It shows high DNA relatedness to serogroup 1 but being serologically distinct from it as well as from other species has been accorded a separate serogroup.

L. parisiensis
The PF-209C-C2 type strain was isolated from cooling tower water from Paris, France in 1981. It autofluoresces bluish-white. In immuno-fluorescence studies it shows minor cross-reaction with *L. bozemanii*, *L. micdadei*, and *L. jordanis*. It shows some DNA relatedness to other bluish-white autofluorescing species.

L. cherrii
The ORW type strain and strains ORB and OR2 were isolated from thermally altered water from Minnesota in 1982. A further strain SC-65-C3 came from a water cistern in the Virgin Islands. These strain autofluoresce bluish-white and show most DNA relatedness to other similar autofluorescing species.

L. steigerwaltii
The SC18-C9 type strain was recovered from tap water from St. Croix, Virgin Islands in 1982. It autofluoresces bluish-white and showed most DNA relatedness to other similar autofluorescing species.

L. santicrucis
The SC-63-C7 type strain was also recovered from tap water from St. Croix, Virgin Islands in 1982. It does not autofluoresce. It showed considerable DNA relatedness to *L. sainthelensii* and less to *L. longbeachae*.

L. israelensis
The Bercovier 4 type strain, an environmental isolate from an oxidation pond in Israel has characteristics of the legionella group though distinct sero-logically from other species.

Morphology

Features of the morphology of legionella species, already discussed in Chapter 1, are best seen in electron micrographs. Characteristically the organisms appear as small coccobacilli, though longer forms can be found. The bacterial surface is smooth or may be convoluted. Sometimes internal globules are evident. Growth is by pinching septate fission (Fig. 2.1(a), (b), (c)). Flagella, single or paired, polar or subpolar are evident particularly during the early growth phase, with short pili around the bacterial surface (Fig. 2.2(a), (b)). In thin section the organisms have a triple unit cell wall

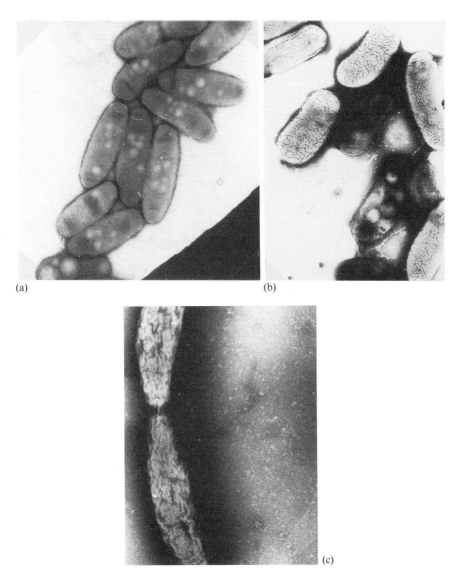

(a)

(b)

(c)

Fig. 2.1 *L. pneumophila* negative stain. (a) Smooth contour, internal globules; original ×20 000. (b) Convoluted surface; original ×40 000. (c) Division by septate fission; original ×40 000. (Electron micrographs kindly provided by Dr F.G. Rodgers.)

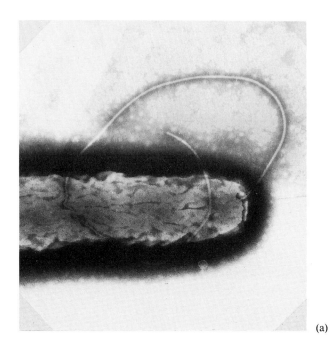

(a)

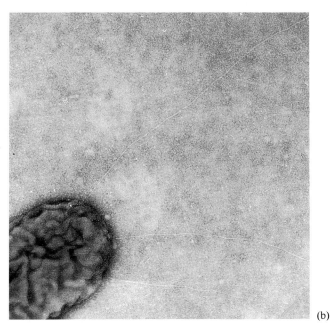

(b)

Fig. 2.2 *L. pneumophila* negative stain. (a) Single polar flagella; original × 66 000. (b) Fine pili on bacterial surface; original × 100 000. (Electron micrographs kindly provided by Dr F.G. Rodgers.)

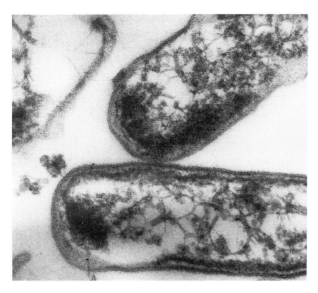

Fig. 2.3 *L. pneumophila* thin section. Triple unit cell wall membrane; original × 115 000. (Electron micrograph kindly provided by Dr F.G. Rodgers.)

membrane, an outer electron-dense layer which may be loose and undulating, an inner less opaque cytoplasmic membrane and an intermediate discontinuous stratum containing peptidoglycan (Fig. 2.3). The bacterial cytoplasm, as with other Gram-negative organisms, contains scattered ribosomes and thread-like nuclear elements (Rodgers 1979, 1983). In the lung of affected patients and in cultured cells, the growth of organisms intracellularly occurs only in the cell cytoplasm.

Phenotypic criteria

Features which are not only characteristic of Legionellaceae but which may aid in distinguishing between them are set out for some of the species in Table 2.4.

Legionellaceae, unusually for Gram-negative bacteria, have a high lipid content including phosphatidylcholine and fatty acids of which more than 80 per cent are branched-chain fatty acids. Extraction of these acids from saponified organisms with analysis by gas liquid chromatography (GLC) has provided distinctive profiles among the species (Edwards and Feltham, 1983; Moss *et al.*, 1977, 1983). Of the total fatty acids of *L. pneumophila*, 85–90 per cent is accounted for by five major acids, the highest concentration being of a saturated branched-chain 16-carbon acid with the methyl branch at the penultimate carbon atom, i-16:0. In decreasing amounts are a monounsaturated 16-carbon straight-chain acid 16:1, a branched chain 15-carbon atom a-15:0, a saturated 14-carbon branched-chain acid i-14:0 and a saturated 17-carbon branched-chain acid a-17:0. Other normal straight-chain saturated acids range from 0–5 per cent (Moss and Dees, 1979(a), (b)).

Table 2.4 Legionella species characteristics

Species	L-cysteine requirement	Motility	Oxidase	Gelatin liquefaction	Starch utilization	Hippurate hydrolysis	Beta-lactamase	Auto-fluorescence (uv light)	Brown pigment on tyrosine YE agar
L. pneumophila	+	+	+/−[x]	+	+	+	+	−[xx]	+
L. bozemanii	+	+	±	+	+	−	+/−	+	+
L. dumoffii	+	+	−	+	NI[xxx]	−	+	+	±
L. micdadei	+	+	+	+	+	−	−	+	−
L. gormanii	+	+	−	+	NI	−	+	+	+
L. longbeachae	+	+	±	+	+	−	+/−	−	+
L. jordanis	+/−	+	+	+	+	−	+	−	+
L. oakridgensis	+/−	−?	−	+	NI	−	±	−	+
L. wadsworthii	+	+	−	+	NI	−	+	−	−
L. feeleii	+	+	−	−	NI	+/−	−	−	±
L. sainthelensi	+	+	+	+	NI	−	+	−	NI

[x] indicates strain variability

[xx] − ranges from nothing to dull yellow, + equals blue-white; in species *L. erythra* and *L. rubrilucens*, not shown, + equals red

[xxx]NI indicates no information

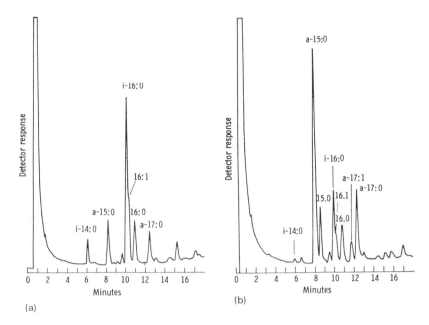

Fig. 2.4 GLC profiles. (a) *L. pneumophila*. (b) *L. micdadei*. (Kindly provided by Richard Edwards.)

Figure 2.4(a) shows the *L. pneumophila* GLC profile and Figure 2.4(b) that of *L. micdadei*.

 L. longbeachae and *L. oakridgensis* also have acid i-16:0 as their main branched-chain fatty acid but other acids such as 16:1 or 16:0 in differing proportions make for distinctive profiles. Among other species including *L. bozemanii*, *L. dumoffii*, *L. gormanii*, *L. micdadei*, *L. jordanis* and *L. wadsworthii* the predominant acid is a saturated branched-chain 15-carbon acid a-15:0 with i-16:0 in a lesser position. *L. micdadei* is distinctive in containing small amounts of a mono-unsaturated branched-chain

Table 2.5 Fatty acids of some legionella species[x]

Fatty acid	*L. pneumophila*	*L. bozemanii*[xx]	*L. micdadei*	*L. longbeachae*	*L. jordanis*
i-14:0	8	4	2	3	2
a-15:0	14	29	39	11	42
i-16:0	32	17	10	19	17
16:0	10	12	9	13	4
16:1	13	11	10	31	7
a-17:0	11	24	25	13	18
a-17:1	2	2	3	2	2
17cyp[xxx]	3	7	2	2	2

[x] These percentage figures of the major distinguishing fatty acids have been compiled from reports, in particular Moss *et al.*, 1977; Moss and Dees 1979a; Hébert *et al.*, 1980; Cherry *et al.*, 1982. Other results may show some deviation

[xx] Approximately similar figures are provided for *L. dumoffii* and *L. gormanii*

[xxx] cyp = cyclopropane acid

17-carbon acid, a-17:1. The cellular fatty acids of recently described species have been stated to qualitatively resemble those of established species (Brenner *et al.*, 1985).

The fatty acid content of some legionella species is shown in Table 2.5. A lack of these cellular fatty acids in various other Gram-negative species confirms the independence of the family Legionellaceae (Edwards and Feltham, 1983). Lipopolysaccharides of *L. pneumophila* show an unusual banding pattern compared with other Gram-negative organisms and are serogroup-specific antigens (Nolte *et al.*, 1986).

Because isoprenoid quinones in bacterial plasma membranes can be of use as chemotaxonomic markers in classification (Collins and Jones, 1981) the detection in legionella species by reverse phase thin layer chromatography of ubiquinones of ten or more isoprene units has afforded additional means of grouping them (Karr *et al.*, 1982). High performance liquid chromatography is also highly successful (Gilbart and Collins, 1985).

In DNA hybridization studies demonstration of a connection between organisms is related to the ability of complementary nucleotides in split single strands of their DNA to recombine and the extent of this recombination reflects the closeness of the relationship. Members of the same species should show a 70 per cent or greater union in tests done at 60°C (Brenner *et al.*, 1978). Within a genus the relationship may be much less exacting.

References

Bercovier, H., Steigerwalt, A.G., Derhi-Cochin, M. *et al.* (1986). Isolation of legionellae from oxidation ponds and fishponds in Israel and description of Legionella israelensis sp. nov. *Int J Syst Bact* **36**, 368–71.

Bibb, W.F., Arnow, P.M., Dellinger, D.L. and Perryman, S.R. (1983). Isolation and characterization of a seventh serogroup of *Legionella pneumophila. J Clin Microbiol* **17**, 346–8.

Bibb, W.F., Sorg, R.J., Thomason, B.M. *et al.* (1981). Recognition of a second serogroup of *Legionella longbeachae. J Clin Microbiol* **14**, 674–7.

Bissett, M.L., Lee, J.O. and Lindquist, D.S. (1983). New serogroup of *Legionella pneumophila*, serogroup 8. *J Clin Microbiol* **17**, 887–91.

Bollin, G.E., Plouffe, J.F., Para, M.F. and Prior, R.B. (1985). Difference in virulence of environmental isolates of *Legionella pneumophila. J Clin Microbiol* **21**, 674–7.

Bozeman, F.M., Humphries, J.W. and Campbell, J.M. (1968). A new group of rickettsia-like agents recovered from guinea pigs. *Acta Virol* **12**, 87–93.

Brenner, D.J., Feeley, J.C. and Feldman, R.A. (1982). Confusion in bacterial nomenclature. *ASM News* **48**, 511–12.

Brenner, D.J., Steigerwalt, A.G., Gorman, G.W. *et al.* (1980). *Legionella bozemanii* sp. Nov. and *Legionella dumoffii* sp. Nov.: Classification of two additional species of *Legionella* associated with human pneumonia. *Curr Microbiol* **4**, 111–16.

Brenner, D.J., Steigerwalt, A.G., Gorman, G.W. *et al.* (1985). Ten new species of *Legionella. Int J Syst Bact* **35**, 50–59.

Brenner, D.J., Steigerwalt, A.G. and McDade, J.E. (1979). Classification of the Legionnaires' disease bacterium: *Legionella pneumophila*, genus novum, species nova of the family Legionellaceae, familia nova. *Ann Intern Med* **90**, 656–8.

Brenner, D.J., Steigerwalt, A.G., Weaver, R.E. *et al.* (1978). Classification of the Legionnaires' disease bacterium: an interim report. *Curr Microbiol* **1**, 71–5.

Brown, A., Vickers, R.M., Elder, E.M. *et al.* (1982). Plasmid and surface antigen markers of endemic and epidemic *Legionella pneumophila* strains. *J Clin Microbiol* **16**, 230–35.

Campbell, J., Bibb, W.F., Lambert, M.A. *et al.* (1984). *Legionella sainthelensi*: a new species of *Legionella* isolated from water near Mt. St. Helens. *Appl Environm Microbiol* **47**, 369–73.

Cherry, W.B., Gorman, G.W., Orrison, L.H. *et al.* (1982). *Legionella jordanis*: a new species of *Legionella* isolated from water and sewage. *J Clin Microbiol* **15**, 290–97.

Christensen, S.W., Tyndall, R.L., Solomon, J.A. *et al.* (1984). Patterns of *Legionella* spp. infectivity in power plant environments and implications for control. In *Legionella: Proceedings of the 2nd International Symposium: Washington, DC.*, pp. 313–15. Edited by Thornsberry, C., Balows, A., Feeley, J.C. and Jakubowski, W. American Society for Microbiology, Washington.

Collins, M.D. and Jones, D. (1981). Distribution of isoprenoid quinone structural types in bacteria and their taxonomic implications. *Microbiol Rev* **45**, 316–54.

Cordes, L.G., Wilkinson, H.W., Gorman, G.W. *et al.* (1979). Atypical Legionella-like organisms: fastidious water-associated bacteria pathogenic for man. *Lancet* **2**, 927–30.

Edelstein, P.H. (1984). Laboratory diagnosis of Legionnaries' disease. In *Legionella: Proceedings of the 2nd International Symposium: Washington, DC.*, pp. 3–5. Edited by Thornsberry, C., Balows, A., Feeley, J.C. and Jakubowski. W. American Society for Microbiology, Washington.

Edelstein, P.H., Bibb, W.F., Gorman, G.W. *et al.* (1984). *Legionella pneumophila* serogroup 9: a cause of human pneumonia. *Ann Intern Med* **101**, 196–8.

Edelstein, P.H., Brenner, D.J., Moss, C.W. *et al.* (1982). *Legionella wadsworthii* species nova; a cause of human pneumonia. *Ann Intern Med* **97**, 809–13.

Edelstein, P.H., McKinney, R.M., Meyer, R.D. *et al.* (1980). Immunologic diagnosis of Legionnaires' disease: cross-reactions with anaerobic and microaerophilic organisms and infections caused by them. *J Infect Dis* **141**, 652–5.

Edelstein, P.H., Meyer, R.D. and Finegold, S.M. (1978). Isolation of a new serotype of Legionnaires' disease bacterium. *Lancet* **2**, 1172–4.

Edelstein, P.H. and Pryor, E.P. (1985). A new biotype of *Legionella dumoffii*. *J Clin Microbiol* **21**, 641–2.

Edwards, R. and Feltham, R.K.A. (1983). Taxonomic implications of the cellular fatty acid content of the Legionellaceae and possibly related species. *FEMS Microbiol Lett* **17**, 251–5.

Elliott, J.A. and Johnson, W. (1981). Immunological and biochemical relationships among flagella isolated from *Legionella pneumophila* serogroups 1, 2 and 3. *Infect Immun* **33**, 602–10.

England, A.C., McKinney, R.M., Skaily, P. and Gorman, G.W. (1980). A fifth serogroup of *Legionella pneumophila*. *Ann Intern Med* **93**, 58–9.

Fliermans C.B., Cherry W.B., Orrison L.H. *et al.* (1981). Ecological distribution of *Legionella pneumophila*. *Appl Environm Microbiol* **41**, 9–16.

Garrity, G.M., Brown, A. and Vickers, R.M. (1980). *Tatlockia* and *Fluoribacter*: two new genera of organisms resembling *Legionella pneumophila*. *Int J System Bact* **30**, 609–14.

Garrity, G.M., Elder, E.M., Davis, B. *et al.* (1982). Serological and genotypic diversity among serogroup 5-reacting environmental *Legionella* isolates. *J Clin Microbiol* **15**, 646–53.

Gilbart, J. and Collins, M.D. (1985). High-performance liquid chromatographic analysis of ubiquinones from new *Legionella* species. *FEMS Microbiol Lett* **26**, 77–82.

Gorman, G.W., Feeley, J.C., Steigerwalt, A.G. *et al.* (1985). *Legionella anisa*: a new species of *Legionella* isolated from potable waters and a cooling tower. *Appl Environm Microbiol* **49**, 305–9.

Hébert, G.A., Steigerwalt, A.G. and Brenner, D.J. (1980). *Legionella micdadei* species nova: classification of a third species of *Legionella* associated with human pneumonia. *Curr Microbiol* **3**, 255–7.

Herwaldt, L.A., Gorman, G.W., McGrath, T. *et al.* (1984). A new *Legionella species, Legionella feeleii*, species nova, causes Pontiac fever in an automobile plant. *Ann Intern Med* **100**, 33–8.

Joly, J.R., Chen, Y-Y. and Ramsay, D. (1983). Serogrouping and subtyping of *Legionella pneumophila* with monoclonal antibodies. *J Clin Microbiol* **18**, 1040–46.

Joly, J.R. and Kenny, G.E. (1982). Antigenic analysis of *Legionella pneumophila* and *Tatlockia micdadei* (*Legionella micdadei*) by two-dimensional (crossed) immuno-electrophoresis. *Infect Immun* **35**, 721–9.

Joly, J.R., McKinney, R.M., Tobin, J.O. *et al.* (1986). Development of a standardized subgrouping scheme for *Legionella pneumophila* serogroup 1 using monoclonal antibodies. *J Clin Microbiol* **23**, 768–71.

Karr, D.E., Bibb, W.F. and Moss, C.W. (1982). Isoprenoid quinones of the genus *Legionella*. *J Clin Microbiol* **15**, 1044–8.

McKinney, R.M., Porschen, R.K., Edelstein, P.H. *et al.* (1981). *Legionella longbeachae* species nova, another etiologic agent of human pneumonia. *Ann Intern Med* **94**, 739–43.

McKinney, R.M., Thacker, L., Harris, P.P. *et al.* (1979). Four serogroups of Legionnaires' disease bacteria defined by direct immunofluorescene. *Ann Intern Med* **90**, 621–4.

McKinney, R.M. Wilkinson, H.W., Sommers, H.M. *et al.* (1980). *Legionella pneumophila* serogroup six: isolation from cases of Legionellosis, identification by immunofluorescence staining, and immunological response to infection. *J Clin Microbiol* **12**, 395–401.

Macrae, A.D., Appleton, P.N. and Laverick, A. (1979). Legionnaires' disease in Nottingham, England. *Ann Intern Med* **90**, 580–83.

Meenhorst, P.L., Reingold, A.L., Groothuis, D.G. *et al.* (1985). Water-related nosocomial pneumonia caused by *Legionella pneumophila* serogroups 1 and 10. *J Infect Dis* **152**, 356–64.

Mitchell, R.G., Pasvol, G. and Newnham, R.S., (1984). Pneumonia due to a *Legionella bozemanii*: first report of a case in Europe. *J Infect Dis* **8**, 251–5.

Morris, G.K., Patton, C.M. Feeley, J.C. *et al.* (1979). Isolation of the Legionnaires' disease bacterium from environmental samples. *Ann Intern Med* **90**, 664–6.

Morris, G.K., Steigerwalt, A., Feeley, J.C. *et al.* (1980). *Legionella gormanii* sp nov. *J Clin Microbiol* **12**, 718–21.

Moss, C.W. and Dees, S.B. (1979a). Further studies of the cellular fatty acid composition of Legionnaires' disease bacteria. *J Clin Microbiol* **9**, 648–9.

Moss, C.W. and Dees, S.B. (1979b). Cellular fatty acid composition of Wiga, a rickettsia-like agent similar to the Legionnaires' disease bacterium. *J Clin Microbiol* **10**, 390–91.

Moss, C.W., Bibb, W.F., Karr, D.E. *et al.* (1983). Cellular fatty acid composition and ubiquinone content of *Legionella feelei* sp. nov. *J Clin Microbiol* **18**, 917–19.

Moss, C.W., Weaver, R.E., Dees, S.B. and Cherry, W.B. (1977). Cellular fatty acid composition of isolates of Legionnaires' disease. *J Clin Microbiol* **6**, 140–43.

Nagington, J., Wreghitt, T.G. and Smith, D.J. (1979) How many Legionnaires? *Lancet* **2**, 536–7.

Nolte, F.S., Conlin, C.A. and Motley, M.A. (1986). Electrophoretic and serological characterization of the lipopolysaccharides of *Legionella pneumophila*. *Infect Immun* **52**, 676–81.

Orrison, L.H., Cherry, W.B., Tyndall, R.L. *et al.* (1983). *Legionella oakridgensis*: unusual new species isolated from cooling tower water. *Appl Environm Microbiol* **45**, 536–45.

Pearlman, E., Engleberg, N.C. and Eisenstein, B.I. (1985). Identification of protein antigens of *Legionella pneumophila* serogroup 1. *Infect Immun* **47**, 74–9.

Rodgers, F.G. (1979). Ultrastructure of *Legionella pneumophila*. *J Clin Pathol* **32**, 1195–202.

Rodgers, F.G. (1983). The role of structure and invasiveness on the pathogenicity of Legionella. *Zbl Bakt Hyg I Abt Orig A* **255**, 138–44.

Rodgers, F.G. and Laverick, T. (1984). *Legionella pneumophila* serogroup 1 flagellar antigen in a passive haemagglutination test to detect antibodies to other *Legionella* species. In *Legionella: Proceedings of the 2nd International Symposium: Washington, DC.*, pp. 42–4. Edited by Thornsberry, C., Balows, A., Feeley, J.C. and Jakubowski, W. American Society for Microbiology, Washington.

Selander, R.K., McKinney, R.M., Whittam, T.S. *et al.* (1985). Genetic structure of populations of *Legionella pneumophila*. *J Bact* **163**, 1021–37.

Sobell, J.D., Krieger, R., Gilpin, R. *et al.* (1983). *Legionella bozemanii*: still another cause of pneumonia. *JAMA* **250**, 383–5.

Tang, P.W., Toma, S., Moss, C.W. *et al.* (1984). *Legionella bozemanii* serogroup 2: a new etiological agent. *J Clin Microbiol* **19**, 30–33.

Taylor, A.G. and Harrison, T.G. (1979). Legionnaires' disease caused by *Legionella pneumophila* serogroup 3. *Lancet* **2**, 47.

Taylor, A.G., Harrison, T.G., Andrews, B.E. and Sillis, M. (1980). Serological differentiation of Legionnaires' disease and *Mycoplasma pneumoniae* pneumonia. *Lancet* **1**, 764.

Thacker, W.L., Wilkinson, H.W. and Benson, R.F. (1983). Comparison of slide agglutination test and direct immunofluorescence assay for identification of *Legionella* isolates. *J Clin Microbiol* **18**, 1113–18.

Thacker, W.L., Wilkinson, H.W., Benson, R.F. *et al.* (1986). 11th serogroup of *Legionella pneumophila* isolated from a patient with fatal pneumonia. *J Clin Microbiol* **23**, 1146–7.

Thacker, W.L., Wilkinson, H.W., Plikaytis, B.B. *et al.* (1985). Second serogroup of *Legionella feeleii* strains isolated from humans. *J Clin Microbiol* **22**, 1–4.

Thomason, B.M. and Bibb, W.F. (1984). Use of absorbed antisera for demonstration of antigenic variation among strains of *Legionella pneumophila* serogroup 1. *J Clin Microbiol* **19**, 794–7.

Tobin, J.O'H., Beare, J., Dunnill, M.S. *et al.* (1980). Legionnaires' disease in a transplant unit: isolation of the causative agent from shower baths. *Lancet* **2**, 118–21.

Watkins, I.D. and Tobin, J.O'H. (1984). Studies with monoclonal antibodies to *Legionella* species. In *Legionella: Proceedings of the 2nd International Symposium: Washington, DC.*, pp. 259–62. Edited by Thornsberry, C., Balows, A., Feeley, J.C. and Jakubowski, W. American Society for Microbiology, Washington.

Watkins, I.D., Tobin J.O'H., Dennis P.J. *et al.* (1985). *Legionella pneumophila* serogroup 1 subgrouping by monoclonal antibodies – an epidemiological tool. *J Hyg, Camb* **95**, 211–16.

Watts, J.C., Hicklin, M.D., Thomason, B.M. *et al.* (1980). Fatal pneumonia caused by *Legionella pneumophila*, serogroup 3: demonstration of the bacilli in extrathoracic organs. *Ann Intern Med* **96**, 186–8.

Wentworth, B.B. and Stiefel, H.E. (1982). Studies of the specificity of Legionella serology. *J Clin Microbiol* **15**, 961–3.

Wilkinson, H.W., Fikes, B.J. and Cruce, D.D. (1979). Indirect immunofluorescence test for serodiagnosis of Legionnaires' disease: evidence for serogroup diversity of Legionnaires' disease bacterial antigens and for multiple specificity of human antibodies. *J Clin Microbiol* **9**, 379-83.

Wilkinson, H.W., Reingold, A.L. Brake, B.J. *et al.* (1983). Reactivity of serum from patients with suspected legionellosis against 29 antigens of Legionellaceae and *Legionella*-like organisms by indirect immunofluorescence assay. *J Infect Dis* **147**, 23-31.

Wilkinson, H.W., Thacker, W.L., Brenner, D.J. and Ryan, K.J. (1985b). Fatal *Legionella maceachernii* pneumonia. *J Clin Microbiol* **22**, 1055.

Wilkinson, H.W., Thacker, W.L., Steigerwalt, A.G. *et al.* (1985a). Second serogroup of *Legionella hackeliae* isolated from a patient with pneumonia. *J Clin Microbiol* **22**, 488-9.

Wong, K.H., Moss, C.W., Hochstein, D.H. *et al.* (1979). 'Endotoxicity' of the Legionnaires' disease bacterium. *Ann Intern Med* **90**, 624-7.

3 Clinical Aspects and Diagnosis of Legionella Infection

The last 100 years have seen an enormous change in the understanding of pneumonia. Prior to the late 1800s, pneumonia was regarded as an inflammation of the lungs related to external and environmental conditions. However, work by Fraenkel and Friedlander in Germany between 1880 and 1884 established the role of bacterial infection in the aetiology of pneumonia. It was rapidly accepted that the majority of pneumonias were caused by bacteria and extensive studies in the first part of the 20th century showed that 90 per cent of pneumonias were due to pneumococcal infection.

With the introduction of antibiotics during the Second World War and their apparent effectiveness in treating pneumonia there was a general loss of interest in the condition. A group of infections that were not typical of pneumococcal infection and which did not respond to penicillin were recognized as the 'atypical' pneumonias. These were caused by *Chlamydia psittaci*, *Coxiella burnetii* and *Mycoplasma pneumoniae*. However, these atypical pneumonias were rarely fatal and were of passing interest to the medical profession.

The dramatic presentation of legionnaires' disease however, in 1976 and the subsequent investigations caught the interest and imagination of the medical profession, the public and the lay press. Since 1976 there has been enormous interest in the problems of not only legionella infection but also in the whole subject of pneumonia.

How common is legionella pneumonia?

It is difficult to be certain how common legionella pneumonia is and there are conflicting reports about this. The answer seems to depend on where, when and how you look for it. In some places it is epidemic and this allows a high local index of suspicion for legionella infection. The classic example of this is at the Wadsworth Medical Centre in Los Angeles where 65 cases of nosocomial legionella pneumonia occurred within 20 months of the hospital opening. Epidemics have also been reported in association with several hospitals, hotels, workplaces and communities in North America and Europe including the major outbreak at Stafford District General Hospital, England in 1985.

Retrospective studies of stored sera or lung tissue from patients with pneumonia have suggested that legionella infection is an uncommon cause of sporadic pneumonia. For example, Foy and colleagues (1979) identified only five cases of legionella infection amongst 500 patients treated for pneumonia in Seattle between 1963 and 1975. The incidence was estimated to be 0.4–2.8/10 000 persons/year. Interpretation of such retrospective figures is obviously difficult because of possible selection bias. Prospective clinical studies of adults have shown the proportions of pneumonias caused by legionella to vary from 0 to 29 per cent. In general, when legionella infection has been sought most actively, the frequency has been higher, but clearly, there must also be a geographical variation (Table 3.1). In Nottingham, England, a study of 127 consecutive adults admitted to hospital with pneumonia (Macfarlane *et al.*, 1982) found pneumococcal pneumonia

Table 3.1 Frequency of legionella pneumonia from various clinical studies from America and Europe

Type of study	Disease studied	Frequency	Location	Reference
Prospective clinical	Pneumonia	22.5 %	Pennsylvania, USA	(Yu *et al.*, 1982)
" "	"	23 %	Chicago, USA	(Carter, 1979)
" "	"	27 %	Denmark	(Friis-Moller *et al.*, 1984)
" "	"	15 %	Nottingham, England	(Macfarlane *et al.*, 1982)
" "	"	2.2 %	Bristol, England	(White *et al.*, 1981)
" "	"	2 %	Multi-centre, Britain	(BTS Research Committee, 1986)
" "	"	6 %	Spain	(Bouza *et al.*, 1984)
" "	"	7.8 %	France	(Mayaud *et al.*, 1984)
" "	Severe pneumonia	10 %	Germany	(Lode *et al.*, 1982)
" "	Lower respiratory infection	1.8 %	Sweden	(Walder *et al.*, 1981)
" "	'Atypical' pneumonia	29 %	Canada	(Marrie *et al.*, 1981)
Retrospective serological	Pneumonia	6.7 %	Scotland	(Fallon, 1982)
"	"	4–11 %	Iowa, USA	(Renner *et al.*, 1979)
"	"	1 %	Seattle, USA	(Foy *et al.*, 1979)
Retrospective Necropsy lung tissue	Pneumonia	7 %	Vermont, USA	(Gerber *et al.*, 1981)
" " "		6.6 %	Ohio, USA	(Fay *et al.*, 1980)

in three-quarters of the patients, but legionella infection was the second commonest cause, occurring in 15 per cent of cases. A repeat study, however, three years later found the proportion had fallen to 5 per cent (Woodhead *et al.*, 1986). Similarly workers in Pittsburgh (Yu *et al.*, 1982) investigated 142 consecutive pneumonia patients specifically looking for legionellosis by serological and cultural methods together with direct fluorescent antibody staining of respiratory secretions and lung tissue. *L. pneumophila* infection was diagnosed in 32 (22.5 per cent) patients and was the commonest single pathogen identified. Two-thirds of the cases were hospital acquired and legionellosis caused 30 per cent of the nosocomial infections. Of the 66 patients with community acquired pneumonia 15 per cent had legionella infection. In contrast, in a six year prospective study from Bristol, it was diagnosed in only three of 210 adults with pneumonia (White *et al.*, 1981) and in a multi-centre hospital based British study of community acquired pneumonia in 1983 it accounted for only 2 per cent of 453 adults (British Thoracic Society Research Committee, 1986).

The conclusion is that legionella infection is an important cause of adult pneumonia in some areas and must be actively considered in patients with both community acquired and also nosocomial pneumonia particularly in those with severe infecction.

Types of legionella infection

Legionella infection manifests in two principal forms, namely legionella pneumonia (legionnaires' disease) or Pontiac fever. It is unclear why these different forms exist or why people similarly exposed may develop either one or the other form of the disease.

A wide range of clinical presentations exist, varying from asymptomatic infection (shown only by sero-conversion), through a mild lower respiratory illness to the rapidly progressive severe pneumonia that many people equate with the classic legionnaires' disease (Haley *et al.*, 1979; Tsai *et al.*, 1979).

Legionella pneumonia

This infection is usually caused by *L. pneumophila* and the clinical, laboratory and radiographic features are well documented. Less commonly, *L. micdadei*, *L. bozemanii*, *L. dumoffii* and other legionella species are implicated and these will be discussed later.

Clinical features of *L. pneumophila* pneumonia

Men are two to three times more frequently affected than women.

Infection in children is rare and the highest incidence is in 40–70 year old people. Persons particularly at risk include smokers, alcoholics, diabetics, those with chronic illness or who are receiving corticosteroids or immuno-suppressive therapy. Seasonal variation in the incidence has been observed in

Table 3.2 Details, symptoms and signs of 739 patients with legionella pneumonia taken from several series (Bouza *et al.*, 1984; Helms *et al.*, 1984; Kirby *et al.*, 1980; Nordstrom *et al.*, 1983; Tsai *et al.*, 1979; Woodhead and Macfarlane, 1985), including data on 297 cases reported to the PHLS Communicable Disease Surveillance Centre, London

	Patients	*No. patients Total No.* with feature/patients reported
Male	73 %	469/641
Current smoker	66 %	235/357
Prior chronic disease		
community acquired	55 %	210/382
nosocomial cases	95 %	81/ 85
Cough	75 %	546/724
New sputum production	45 %	292/656
Dyspnoea	50 %	373/739
Chest pain	36 %	270/739
Haemoptysis	21 %	75/356
Rigors	59 %	187/316
Myalgias	38 %	267/693
Upper respiratory symptoms	13 %	22/166
Headache	32 %	129/399
Confusion	45 %	294/644
Any neurological symptoms	45 %	115/253
Nausea/vomiting	30 %	185/614
Diarrhoea	33 %	221/661
Abdominal pain	8 %	28/350
Fever above 39°C	70 %	236/338
Relative bradycardia	40 %	72/179
Bronchial breathing in lung	16 %	44/270
Crepitations in lung	74 %	210/284

several countries; in the UK, most cases occur in the summer and autumn. Sometimes there is a history of a recent holiday abroad or a stay in hospital.

There are no unique clinical and laboratory features of legionella pneumonia and it frequently presents like any other lobar pneumonia. Common features are summarized in Table 3.2. Typically, after an incubation period of 2–10 days, the illness starts fairly abruptly with high fever, rigors, headache and myalgia. Upper respiratory tract symptoms are often absent. A skin rash is rare (Allen *et al*, 1985; Woodhead and Macfarlane, 1985). The cough that follows may be minimal and dry but small amounts of purulent sputum may appear after 3–4 days. Some haemoptysis occurs in about a quarter of cases. Dyspnoea and respiratory distress are common. The illness often progresses quickly, requiring hospital admission within 3–6 days after disease onset. By a week, nearly 80 per cent of patients are under medical care (Helms *et al.*, 1984).

The patients usually look ill and toxic and have a high fever. Temperatures of 39.5°C or more are found in two-thirds to three-quarters of cases and 60 per cent have a relative bradycardia. Herpes labialis is uncommon and its presence is suggestive of pneumococcal pneumonia, being found in 30 per cent of such cases. Focal crepitations are heard in the chest in over 80 per cent of cases; bronchial breathing is present in less than 20 per cent. Sometimes non-respiratory problems such as diarrhoea or confusion and delirium may dominate the clinical picture and mask the true diagnosis of pneumonia. The liver may be palpable or tender. Splenomegaly and generalized lymphadeno-pathy are not features in reported clinical series although enlarged spleens were found in over half of the cases in one pathological study (Weisenburger *et al.*, 1981).

Laboratory features

A wide variety of laboratory abnormalities have been reported in patients with legionella pneumonia. The total white cell count is only moderately raised to between 10 000 and 20 000 per mm³ in a half to three-quarters of patients and 15 per cent or less have levels of more than 20 000 per mm³ (Beaty, 1984; Davis *et al.*, 1982; Helms *et al.*, 1984; Woodhead and Macfarlane, 1985). The erythrocyte sedimentation rate is usually raised; cold agglutinins are unusual (Kirby *et al.*, 1980; Tsai *et al.*, 1979). Some abnormality of liver function is detected in two-thirds to three-quarters of patients but frank jaundice is rare (Kirby *et al.*, 1980; Macfarlane, 1983). Hyponatraemia is a common finding in association with acute legionella pneumonia, occurring in about a half of all cases (Davis *et al.*, 1981; Miller, 1982; Woodhead and Macfarlane, 1985). Various reasons for this have been suggested. Inappropriate secretion of antidiuretic hormone has been impli-cated in some cases (Kirby *et al.*, 1980). It appears that hypovolaemia may also be important. The body responds to hypovolaemia by conserving cir-culating volume through the appropriate secretion of antidiuretic hormone. Hypovolaemia may arise from reduced oral intake, sweating, high fever, toxaemia, nausea and diarrhoea. Simultaneous blood and urine electrolyte estimations in 19 adults with hyponatraemia from different pneumonias, including legionella pneumonia, revealed that a high urinary sodium (as found in the syndrome of inappropriate secretion of antidiuretic hormone) appears to be the exception rather than the rule (Macfarlane and Ward, 1982).

Proteinuria is common, and unexplained haematuria on initial urinalysis was found in 40 per cent of patients during the original epidemic in Philadelphia. Although haematuria has been noted commonly in other studies (Woodhead and Macfarlane, 1986a), it has not been a common fea-ture in a large number of patients (Kirby *et al.*, 1980). Some abnormality of blood urea and creatinine is sometimes seen during the acute illness but overt renal failure is relatively uncommon.

If sputum is produced, it generally looks mucoid. A Gram stain char-acteristically shows scanty neutrophils and no predominant microorga-nism. On occasions the Gram stain can be helpful in diagnosis (Baptiste–Desruisseaux *et al.*, 1985). Routine sputum and blood cultures will be negative for the usual respiratory pathogens, unless a mixed infection is present. If pleural fluid is detected and sampled, it will usually be an exudate with some neutrophils present but no pathogens identified on staining or culture (Kirby *et al.*, 1980). Such negative results on routine micro-biological tests should always raise the suspicion of legionella infection, particularly if antibiotics have not been given before the specimens have been taken.

Radiographic features

The chest radiograph can occasionally be normal when the patient first presents, but nearly all will have changes. In one study of nosocomial legionella
pneumonia the radiographs obtained on the first day of symptoms, were
abnormal in 21 of 24 patients. Infiltrates appeared in the other three by the
third day of the illness (Kirby *et al.*, 1979). The initial type of shadowing is
variable. In a review of 70 cases, the initial radiograph showed lobar and seg-
mental shadowing in a third, diffuse patchy shadowing in a third and poorly
marginated rounded shadows in the remainder. In this study, the delay
between onset of symptoms and the first radiograph was on average 3 days
(Fairbank *et al.*, 1983). In a study of 49 adults with community acquired
legionella pneumonia presenting 6 days after the start of symptoms, 82 per
cent showed mainly homogeneous shadowing and the rest had patchy
shadows (Macfarlane *et al.*, 1984). The lower lobes are affected most
commonly as with any pneumonia. On presentation, more than one lobe is
involved in only a third to a half of all cases.

Deterioration of the chest radiograph after presentation is particularly
common with legionella pneumonia (Fig. 3.1(a), (b), (c) and (d)) and is seen
in two-thirds of cases. This may happen in spite of apparently effective antimicrobial therapy. Either there may be spread of the shadowing within a
particular lobe to give homogeneous lobar shadowing, or spread to a
contiguous lobe. Involvement of the opposite lung occurs in a quarter of
cases (Kirby *et al.*, 1979; Macfarlane *et al.*, 1984). Pleural effusions can be
detected in a quarter to a half of cases but these are usually small and rarely
occupy more than a third of the hemithorax. Sometimes they may be due to
underlying cardiac failure. The ability to detect pleural fluid can be improved
by using lateral decubitus radiographs. Some degree of pulmonary collapse is
not uncommon and although it can be due to significant endobronchial
obstruction (e.g. neoplasm, foreign body) it also occurs in otherwise uncom-
plicated pneumonias including legionella infection. Hilar lymphadenopathy
is a very unusual finding on the radiograph although enlarged carinal and
hilar nodes are found at necropsy (Kirby *et al.*, 1980). Lung cavitation is
unusual except in patients who are immunosuppressed (Bouza *et al.*, 1984;
Fairbank *et al.*, 1983; Hughes and Anderson, 1985; Kirby *et al.*, 1979).
Secondary infection by other pathogens have been implicated in some of
these cases of cavitation.

Legionella pneumonia is peculiar in showing a slow rate of radiographic
resolution in survivors. This may lag considerably behind clinical recovery.
This slow radiographic resolution is well documented (Fairbank *et al.*, 1983)
and is unusual in other forms of community acquired pneumonia except for
bacteraemic pneumococcal pneumonia (Macfarlane *et al.*, 1984). The rate of
resolution of pneumonia is also affected by increasing age and the presence of
underlying chronic lung disease. The slow rate of resolution may raise the
possibility of an underlying bronchial obstruction from lung cancer and
legionella pneumonia has been diagnosed retrospectively in some patients
referred for bronchoscopy for this reason (Miller and Smith, 1978). Only one
series has reported fairly rapid clearance of radiographic shadowing. Kirby
and colleagues (1979) found radiographic resolution for three-quarters of 21

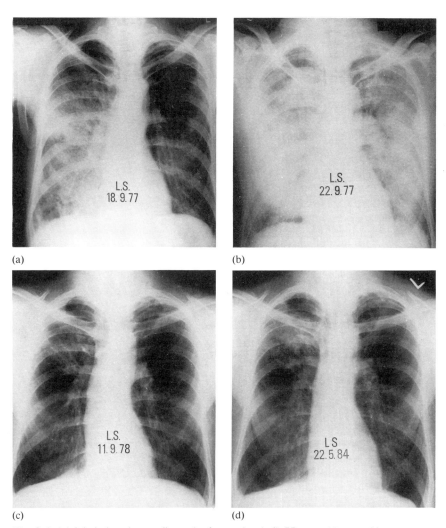

Fig. 3.1 (a) Admission chest radiograph of a previously fit 55-year old man with
L. pneumophila pneumonia. (b) Four days later marked deterioration with spread of shadows
to all lobes. Patient required assisted ventilation. (c) Same patient, 1 year later. Feeling
perfectly well but radiograph shows persistent shadows and contraction of right upper lobe.
(d) Nearly 7 years later after pneumonia marked contraction and fibrosis of right upper lobe;
confirmed on tomography.

survivors of legionella pneumonia within two months. However, these
patients were diagnosed and treated rapidly during an outbreak of hospital
nosocomial infection. The reason for the slow resolution is not clear. The
presence of intrapulmonary, irregular and linear streaky shadows that persist
after resolution of pulmonary consolidation, suggests that recovery may
involve fibrosis or persisting atalectasis (see Fig. 3.1). Pathological studies in
animals support the view that lung fibrosis is common following infection
(Baskerville, 1984).

Table 3.3 Some comparative radiographic features of different types of community acquired pneumonia adapted from Macfarlane *et al.*, 1984; Macfarlane and Macrae, 1983

	Legionella pneumonia	Pneumococcal pneumonia	Mycoplasma pneumonia	Psittacosis
Mainly homogeneous shadows	82 %	74 %	50 %	60%
Unilobe involvement at presentation	61 %	61 %	48 %	60 %
Pleural effusions	24 %	34 %	20 %	20 %
Hilar lymphadenopathy	0 %	0 %	22 %	0 %
Lung cavitation	2 %	4 %	0 %	10 %
Radiographic deterioration during treatment	65 %	32 %	25 %	0 %
% with normal ⋅ radiograph after 8 weeks	35 %	60 %	90 %	60 %

Some comparative radiographic features of common types of community acquired pneumonia are shown in Table 3.3. There are no unique radiographic features of legionella pneumonia sufficiently distinct to differentiate it from other types, but the most characteristic features include radiographic deterioration after presentation and delayed resolution in survivors.

Complications

Complications affecting nearly every system of the body have been reported with legionella infection (Woodhead and Macfarlane, 1985). These may arise either from a multi-system toxic effect or from direct spread of the infection by lymphatic and haematogenous pathways to other organs of the body. No specific exotoxin has been identified to date and detection of infection in other parts of the body is being increasingly reported, although accompanying pathological changes are minimal. Legionella bacteria have been occasionally cultured from the blood (Edelstein *et al.*, 1979; Macrae *et al.*, 1979; Martin *et al.*, 1984) and metastatic foci have been found in such diverse sites as the bone marrow (Humayun *et al.*, 1981), the colon (Fogliani *et al.*, 1982), the appendix (Holt, 1981), the kidney (Dorman *et al.*, 1980) pleural (Muder *et al.*, 1984) and pericardial fluids (Maycock *et al.*, 1983), brain and liver (Cutz *et al.*, 1982). Direct fluorescent antibody studies have identified bacteria in the liver, spleen and mediastinal lymph nodes of patients who have died (Evans *et al.*, 1981; Watts *et al.*, 1980). Arterio-venous fistula infection has been reported in two patients with chronic renal failure suffering from legionella pneumonia (Kalweit *et al.*, 1982).

Pulmonary complications
Acute respiratory failure is the most important immediate complication to recognize. Assisted ventilation has been required in 11–46 per cent of hospitalized patients (Beaty, 1984; Davis *et al.*, 1981; Woodhead and

Macfarlane, 1986). This should be started early, as the prognosis in such patients is not hopeless and over 50 per cent will survive. Death in such cases is usually due to shock and circulatory collapse rather than uncorrectable hypoxia. Pulmonary complications that are occasionally seen include pneumothorax, lung abscesses, empyemas and prolonged impairment of lung function. In a number of patients, reduced diffusing capacity has been observed 2 years after recovery from the pneumonia (Lattimer *et al.*, 1979). Obliterative bronchiolitis has been reported (Sato *et al.*, 1985).

Cardiac complications

Cardiac complications are well recognized (Nelson *et al.*, 1984). Acute peri-carditis has been reported, together with pericardial effusions (Durand *et al.*, 1984; Harris, 1981). In one case pericardial constriction developed and required pericardectomy. Pericarditis may occur without pneumonia (Nelson *et al.*, 1985). Clinical and laboratory findings of myocardial involve-ment, causing overt cardiac failure and reversible myocarditis have been reported in a few adults and children (Gross *et al.*, 1981; Pastoris *et al.*, 1984). There is one well documented case of *L. pneumophila* endocarditis, on a prosthetic valve (McCabe *et al.*, 1984). This was controlled by removal of the infected valve. Interestingly there was no pneumonia or infection elsewhere. Endocarditis on a native valve has not been proven although it has been sus-pected (Finegold, 1984). Mild hypotension is common but true shock is unusual and carries a poor prognosis.

Neuromuscular complications

A wide variety of neurological complications have been reported, occurring in about a third of cases (Johnson *et al.*, 1984). The most common manifesta-tions of central nervous system involvement are headache, confusion and delirium suggesting a diffuse encephalopathy. Delirium unrelated to hypoxia or metabolic disturbance may lead the clinician to diagnose delirium tremens even in the absence of a history of alcohol abuse. Meningitis is not seen. Where cerebrospinal fluid has been sampled it has invariably been normal. More serious neurological complications include acute brain stem and cerebellar ataxia (Baker *et al.*, 1981; Maskill and Jordan, 1981; Nigro *et al.*, 1983; Pearson and Dadds, 1981), peripheral neuropathy (Holliday *et al.*, 1982; Morgan and Gawler, 1981), neurogenic bladder dysfunction (Bernardini *et al.*, 1985), chorea (Bamford and Hakin, 1982) and Guillain-Barré syndrome (Marthedal and Fisch-Thomsen, 1981). Such complications are not always reversible and cerebellar ataxia and retrograde amnesia can persist for many months. Significant elevation of skeletal muscle enzymes have been encountered in a high proportion of cases. This has been associated with histological evidence of rhabdomyolysis in a few instances (Beaty, 1984). The frequency of neuromuscular problems has led to the suggestion of a specific neurotoxin in legionella infection (Kennedy *et al.*, 1981). However, confusion and raised skeletal muscle creatine kinase isoenzymes are also found in other severe pneumonias (Macfarlane *et al.*, 1982).

Renal complications

Although abnormalities of serum electrolytes and urine examination are not unusual, overt renal failure requiring active therapy is uncommon (Fenves, 1985). In some instances renal failure has been related to shock and acute tubular necrosis (Oredugba *et al.*, 1980; Williams *et al.*, 1980). Reversible interstitial nephritis (Poulter *et al.*, 1981) and glomerulo-nephritis (Saleh *et al.*, 1980 Wegmuller *et al.*, 1985) have also been documented. Acute renal failure from myoglobinuria is well recorded and is usually, but not always, reversible (Hall *et al.*, 1983; Johnson and Etter, 1984; Kerr *et al.*, 1978; Posner *et al.*, 1980). In survivors, persisting renal impairment is uncommon. Legionella infection can precipitate rejection of a transplant kidney on occasions (Kirby *et al.*, 1980).

Other complications

There have been isolated reports of arthritis (Loveridge, 1981), hypoplastic anaemia (Hajiroussou and Joshi, 1980), autoimmune haemolytic anaemia (Strikas *et al.*, 1983), thrombocytopaenic purpura with immune complex formation (Riggs *et al.*, 1982), skin rashes (Anderson *et al.*, 1981; Helms *et al.*, 1981), pancreatitis (Arneborn and Kallings, 1985; Gordon *et al.*, 1980), sinusitis (Schlanger *et al.*, 1984) and cutaneous abscess (Ampel *et al.*, 1985) associated with legionella infection.

Prolonged sequelae

Although individual case reports have noted permanent sequelae following legionella pneumonia, there are unfortunately no properly controlled follow up studies of the rate of recovery and incidence of prolonged sequelae in survivors.

Johnson *et al.*, (1984) reviewed reported neurological complications and noted that ten of the 52 cases with cerebellar dysfunction had prolonged sequelae and three had persistent memory loss. Of 68 patients reported in a Swedish outbreak (Nordstrom *et al.*, 1983) four had protracted muscle pain or weakness. Others have reported survivors taking up to three months to lose feelings of lethargy and malaise (Jenkins *et al.*, 1979). Two years after the Philadelphia outbreak, 18 of 31 patients complained of tiredness, 13 were dyspnoeic and eight had myalgias and arthralgias. However, lack of a control group and patients' knowledge of their disease make sensible interpretation of these results difficult. Radiographic follow up studies have shown persisting abnormalities on the chest radiograph in a quarter or more of survivors, but these are probably rarely of functional significance (Fairbank *et al.*, 1983; Macfarlane *et al.*, 1984).

The overall impression is that although recovery may take several weeks, the large majority of survivors are left without any clinical disability.

Legionella pneumonia in children

Reports of legionella infection in children are uncommon. A one year prospective study of 206 children hospitalized with pneumonia identified only two possible cases of legionella infection: in a 15 month old girl and a six year old boy (Orenstein *et al.*, 1981). Case reports of infection in both healthy (Helms *et al.*, 1984; Millunchick *et al.*, 1981; Simpson *et al.*, 1980) and immunosuppressed (Kovatch *et al.*, 1984; Ryan *et al.*, 1979) children are recorded. Infection may present in atypical ways. Serological studies on 66 children presenting with various acute neurological disorders identified three cases with significant antibody rises to legionellae, all in children with acute cerebellar ataxia. All recovered quickly, two having received oral dexamethasone (Nigro *et al.*, 1983). Similarly arrhythmias and myocarditis have been associated with legionella infection in children without pneumonia (Pastoris *et al.*, 1985).

Infections by other legionella species

The majority of legionella infections have been caused by *L. pneumophila*, usually serogroup 1. Species identified in sporadic cases of legionellosis in the United States over the last few years have shown 69 per cent caused by *L. pneumophila* serogroup 1, 18 per cent by other *L. pneumophila* serogroups, 8 per cent by *L. micdadei*, and 4 per cent by *L. bozemanii* or *L. longbeachae* (Kuritsky *et al.*, 1984). However, comparative studies have revealed no significant differences in the the clinical presentation of patients with these various legionella infections (Beaty, 1984).

L. micdadei is the commonest of the other legionella species to cause pneumonia and has been identified as a possible aetiological agent in approximately 1 per cent of pneumonias from various studies (Broome, 1984). Commonly *L. micdadei* pneumonia is a nosocomial infection most likely to develop in severely immunocompromised patients or those recovering from surgery (Muder *et al.*, 1983). In one hospital outbreak 25 of 26 patients affected by *L. micdadei* were immunocompromised and the mortality was 30 per cent. When 101 consecutive kidney transplant recipients were studied in the Presbyterian University Hospital in Pittsburgh for the development of nosocomial legionellosis, the interval from transplant to onset of pneumonia was shorter for patients developing *L. micdadei* pneumonia than for patients with *L. pneumophila* pneumonia. This suggested that the former infection occurred when the recipients were more immunocompromised (Rudin *et al.*, 1984). Cases of *L. dumoffii* infections (Stamenkovic *et al.*, 1983) and community acquired *L. micdadei* and *L. bozemanii* pneumonia have occasionally been reported from Europe (Macfarlane *et al.*, 1982; Mitchell *et al.*, 1984).

Legionellae and other respiratory pathogens – mixed infections

Dual infections with *L. pneumophila* serogroup 1 and *L. micdadei* have been described in a total of seven patients from one institution. These patients had a severe pneumonia and four died (Muder *et al.*, 1983, 1984). Nearly all were markedly immunocompromised. There are reports of mixed infections between *L. pneumophila* and viral infections (Helms *et al.*, 1984), *Mycobacterium tuberculosis* (Milder and Rough, 1982), *Mycoplasma pneumoniae* (Helms *et al.*, 1984), *Coxiella burnetii* (Domaradzki *et al.*,1984), *Klebsiella species* (Kirby *et al.*, 1980) and *Streptococcus pneumoniae*

(Macfarlane *et al.*, 1982). The possibility of a mixed infection should be considered if a patient is not improving as expected.

Comparative features of community acquired and nosocomial legionella pneumonia

The clinical findings of nosocomial and community acquired forms are very similar both for sporadic (Helms *et al.*, 1984; Woodhead and Macfarlane, 1986a) and epidemic cases (Kirby *et al.*, 1980). The main difference is that underlying disease is far commoner in the patients with nosocomial pneumonia compared with those with infections acquired in the community. The features of the pneumonia may also be modified by the underlying illness. In one series 61 per cent of community acquired cases had an underlying disease compared with 100 per cent for the nosocomial cases (Helms *et al.*, 1984). The latter figure is hardly surprising as all the patients are in hospital because of illness in the first place. The importance of underlying host factors is well shown by the epidemic at the Veterans Administration Wadsworth Medical Centre in Los Angeles when nosocomial legionella pneumonia became common in patients but rarely affected similarly exposed but healthy hospital employees and medical staff (Kirby *et al.*, 1980).

Corticosteroid and immunosuppression are major risk factors. They may be associated with 90 per cent of nosocomial cases compared with only 14 per cent of community acquired pneumonias. Renal transplant recipients seemed particularly prone to legionella infection (Helms *et al.*, 1984; Kirby *et al.*, 1980). In such immunocompromised patients, the infection is more severe and more frequently lethal than in the general population, with mortality rates up to 30–50 per cent (Davis *et al.*, 1981). In a comparative study from the University of Ohio the case fatality rate for nosocomial infection was 70 per cent compared with 22 per cent for community acquired disease (Helms *et al.*, 1984). In this study, however, only four in the former group had received erythromycin, compared with 31 in the latter.

Differentiation of legionella infection from other pneumonias

Earlier reports suggested that legionella pneumonia was associated with a distinctive clinical, laboratory and radiographic pattern that allowed early differentiation from other pneumonias. However, it is now generally agreed that there is a broad overlap with other types of pneumonia and that there are no distinguishing features that can be relied on to identify sporadic cases of legionella infection (Beaty, 1984; Woodhead and Macfarlane, 1986b). In an epidemic situation, however, some of the features of legionella pneumonia may be sufficiently distinct to differentiate it from other types of nosocomial infection. Important clues suggesting legionella pneumonia include high fever, unexplained confusion, multi-system involvement (e.g. central nervous system, gastro-intestinal system, liver, renal, heart and skeletal muscle involvement), sparse and mucoid sputum with scanty pus cells on staining and no predominant pathogens on culture and also a lack of response to beta lactam and aminoglycoside antibiotics.

Community acquired pneumonias that can produce a very similar clinical picture to legionella infection include Q fever, psittacosis and pneumococcal infection, particularly when complicated by bacteraemia. Mycoplasma pneumonia tends to affect younger people who give a longer history of illness and have less evidence of multi-system involvement. Total white cell counts tend to be higher in other bacterial pneumonias, only moderately raised in legionella infections and near normal in atypical and viral pneumonias. Some epidemiological clues may be obtained from the history. Legionella pneumonia is far commoner in the summer months and may be associated with a recent hospital stay or holiday in a large hotel. Viral and pneumococcal pneumonias are commoner in the winter months. A history of contact with exotic birds or fowl may suggest psittacosis and contact with farm animals or their excreta should raise the possibility of Q fever. Mycoplasma pneumonia occurs in epidemics every 3 years or so and suspicion should be heightened during such periods. The presence of raised cold agglutinins or a positive bedside cold agglutinin screening test (positive in over 50 per cent cases of mycoplasma pneumonia) strengthens this possibility (Macfarlane and Neale, 1979).

Pontiac fever

This is the acute non-pneumonic form of legionella infection. It gets its name from the explosive epidemic of a flu-like illness that occurred in a County Health Department building in Pontiac, Michigan in 1968. Subsequent studies in 1978 confirmed that this illness was caused by *L. pneumophila* bacterium (Glick *et al.*, 1978). Since then several outbreaks have been described involving *L. pneumophila* serogroup 1 and 6 and also a recently described, legionella species *Legionella feeleii* (Broome, 1984; Herwaldt *et al.*, 1984). Why legionella infection should manifest itself either as legionella pneumonia, with a low attack rate and a significant mortality, or as Pontiac fever, often with a very high attack rate and no mortality, has not been fully explained. Isolates of *L. pneumophila* associated with both types of illness have shown no difference in virulence in animal models (Huebner *et al.*, 1984) but the use of monoclonal antibody tests may show up strain differences (Joly and Winn, 1984).

Features of Pontiac fever

Pontiac fever presents as an acute, short-lived, self-limiting, febrile illness. It may be this form of the disease which accounts for much of the seropositivity found in the general population (Glick *et al.*, 1978). For instance, there was a significant association between seropositivity and a flu-like illness, for staff tested during the legionella outbreak at Stafford District General Hospital, England (Committee of Inquiry, 1986).

The clinical picture found in the original outbreak in Pontiac summarizes the usual presentation and findings (Table 3.4). The attack rate is very high

Table 3.4 Features of Pontiac fever adapted from Glick *et al.*, 1978

Fever	86 %
Rigors	83 %
Myalgias	95 %
Headache	88 %
Cough	46 %
Chest ache	55 %
Vomiting	10 %
Diarrhoea	21 %
Confusion	19 %
Unsteadiness	12 %
Dizziness	51 %

(95 per cent of those staff exposed in the Pontiac outbreak) and usually affects previously healthy people. The incubation period varies from 4–66 hours but is usually 36–48 hours. There is an abrupt onset of flu-like symptoms with only modest respiratory complaints (Table 3.4). Examination reveals a tachycardia and high fever, usually greater than 39.5°C, but no localizing signs in the chest. Apart from a slight polymorphonuclear leucocytosis, haemotological, biological and microbiological tests are normal or negative, as is the chest radiograph. The illness resolves spontaneously, usually within 2–5 days and deaths have not been reported. Some patients experience non-specific symptoms and lassitude for much longer. One unusual feature of the original outbreak was a recurrent illness in 14 per cent of the employees who were re-exposed to the building within a few days of recovering from the original illness. The clinical diagnosis is usually made retrospectively by serological testing and treatment is symptomatic.

References

Allen, T.P., Fried, J.S., Wiegmann, T.B., *et al.* (1985). Legionnaires' disease associated with rash and renal failure. *Arch Intern Med* **145**, 729–30.

Ampel, N.M., Ruben, F.L. and Norden, C.W. (1985). Cutaneous abscess caused by *Legionella micdadei* in an immunosuppressed patient. *Ann Intern Med* **102**, 630–32.

Anderson, R., Bergan, T., Halvorsen, K., *et al.* (1981). Legionnaires' disease combined with erythema multiforme in a 3 year old boy. *Acta Paediatrica Scandinavica* **70**, 427–30.

Arneborn, P. and Kallings, I. (1985). Acute pancreatitis possibly caused by *Legionella micdadei. Scand J Infec Dis* 17, 229–31.

Baker, P.C., Price, T.R. and Allen, C.D. (1981). Brain stem and cerebellar dysfunction with Legionnaires' disease. *J Neurol, Neurosurg and Psychiat* **44**, 1054–6.

Bamford, J.M. and Hakin, R.N. (1982). Chorea after legionnaires' disease. *Br Med J* **284**, 1232.

Baptiste-Desruisseaux, D., Duperval, R. and Marcoux, J.A. (1985). Legionnaires' disease in the immunocompromised host: usefulness of Gram's stain. *Can Med Assocn J* 133, 117–18.

Baskerville, A. (1984). Summary of pathology and pathophysiology in legionella. In *Legionella Proceedings of the 2nd International Symposium*, Washington, DC., pp. 136–41. Edited by Thornsberry, C., Balows, A., Feeley, J.C. and Jakubowski, W. American Society for Microbiology, Washington.

Beaty, H.N. (1984). Clinical features of legionellosis. In *Legionella*: *Proceedings of the 2nd International Symposium, Washington, DC.*, pp. 6–10. Edited by Thornsberry, C., Balows, A., Feeley, J.C. and Jakubowski, W. American Society for Microbiology, Washington.

Bernardini, D.L., Lerrick, K.S., Hoffman, K. and Lange, M. (1985). Neurogenic bladder. New clinical finding in Legionnaires' disease. *Am J Med* **78**, 1045–6.

Bouza, E. and Rodriguez-Creixems, M. (1984). Legionnaires' disease in Spain. In *Legionella*: *Proceedings of the 2nd International Symposium, Washington, DC.*, pp. 15–17. Edited by Thornsberry, C., Balows, A., Feeley, J.C. and Jakubowski, W. American Society for Microbiology, Washington.

British Thoracic Society Research Committee. (1986). Community acquired pneumonia in adults in British Hospitals in 1982–3: A BTS/PHLS survey of aetiology, mortality, prognostic factors and outcome. *QJM*. In press.

Broome, C.V. (1984). Current issues in epidemiology of Legionellosis. In *Legionella*: *Proceedings of the 2nd International Symposium, Washington, DC.*, pp. 205–9. Edited by Thornsberry, C., Balows, A., Feeley, J.C. and Jakubowski, W. American Society for Microbiology, Washington.

Carter, J.B. (1979). Legionnaires' disease at a community hospital. *Ann Intern Med* **91**, 794.

Committee of Inquiry (1986). First Report of the Committee of Inquiry into the Outbreak of Legionnaires' Disease in Stafford in April 1985, London, p. 22. HMSO, London.

Cutz, E., Thorner, P.S., Rao, C.P., *et al.* (1982). Disseminated *Legionella pneumophila* infection in an infant with severe combined immunodeficiency. *J Pediatr* **100**, 760–62.

Davis, G.S., Winn, W.C. and Beaty, H.N. (1981). Legionnaires' disease. *Clin Chest Med* **2**, 145–66.

Domaradzki, M.D., Hausser, J.L. and Gosselin, F. (1984). Coexistence of Legionnaires' disease and Q fever in a single patient. *Can Med Assocn J* **130**, 1022–3.

Dorman, S.A., Hardin, N.J. and Winn, W.C. (1980). Pyelonephritis associated with *Legionella pneumophila* serogroup 4. *Ann Intern Med* **93**, 835–7.

Durand, S., Damecour, C. and Jacotot, B. (1984). A case of Legionnaires' disease with pericardial involvement. *Nouvelle Presse Medicale* **13**, 1516.

Edelstein, P.H., Meyer, R.D. and Finegold, S.M. (1979). Isolation of *Legionella pneumophila* from blood. *Lancet* **1**, 750–51.

Evans, C.P. and Winn, W.C. (1981). Extrathoracic localisation of *Legionella pneumophila* in Legionnaires' pneumonia. *Am J Clin Pathol* **79**, 813–15.

Fairbank, J.T. Mamourian, A.C., Dietrich, P.A. and Girod, J.C. (1983). The chest radiograph in Legionnaires' disease. *Radiology* **147**, 33–4.

Fay, D., Baird, I.M., Aguirre A., *et al.* (1980). Unrecognised Legionnaires' disease as a cause of fatal illness. *JAMA* **243**, 2311–13.

Fallon, R.J. (1982). Legionella infections in Scotland. *J Hyg* **89**, 439–48.

Fenves, A.Z. (1985). Legionnaires' disease associated with acute renal failure: a report of two cases and review of the literature. *Clin Nephrol* **23**, 96–100.

Finegold, S.M. (1984). Clinical features and laboratory diagnosis. In *Legionella*: *Proceedings of the 2nd International Symposium.*, Washington, DC., pp. 49–52. Edited by Thornsberry, C., Balows, A., Feeley, J.C. and Jakubowski, W. American Society for Microbiology, Washington.

Fogliani, J., Domenget, J.T., Hohn, B., *et al.* (1982). Legionnaires' disease with digestive tract lesions. One case. *Nouvelle Presse Medicale* **11**, 2699–702.

Foy, H.M., Hayes, P.S., Cooney, M.K., *et al.* (1979). Legionnaires' disease in a prepaid medical case group in Seattle 1963–75. *Lancet* **1**, 767–70.

Friis-Moller, A., Rechnitzek, C., Black, F.T., *et al.* (1984). In *Legionella*:

Proceedings of the 2nd International Symposium, Washington, DC., pp. 258–9. Edited by Thornsberry, C., Balows, A., Feeley, J.C. and Jakubowski, W. American Society for Microbiology, Washington.

Gerber, J.E., Casey, C.A., Martin, P. and Winn, W.C. (1981). Legionnaires' disease in Vermont, 1972–1976. *Am J Clin Pathol* **76**, 816–18.

Glick, T.H., Gregg, M.B., Berman, B., *et al.* (1978). Pontiac fever. An epidemic of unknown aetiology in a health department: I. Clinical and epidemiologic aspects. *Am J Epidemiol* **107**, 149–60.

Gordon, V., Postic, B., Zmyslinski, R.W. and Khan, A.H. (1980). Legionnaires' disease complicated by acute pancreatitis: case report. *Mil Med* **145**, 345–7.

Gross, D., Willens, H. and Zeldis, S.M. (1981). Myocarditis in Legionnaires' disease. *Chest* **79**, 232–4.

Hajiroussou, V.J. and Joshi, R.C. (1980). Hypoplastic anaemia associated with Legionnaires' disease. *Br Med J* **280**, 366–7.

Haley, C.E., Cohen, M.L., Halter, J. and Mayer, R.D. (1979). Nosocomial Legionnaires' disease. A continuing common source epidemic at Wadsworth Medical Centre. *Ann Intern Med* **90**, 583–6.

Hall, S.L., Wasserman, M., Dall, L. and Schubert, T. (1983). Acute renal failure secondary to myoglobinurea associated with Legionnaires' disease. *Chest* **84**, 633–5.

Harris, L.F. (1981). Legionnaires' disease associated with massive pericardial effusion. *Arch Intern Med* **141**, 1385.

Helms, C.M., Johnson, W., Donaldson, M.F. and Corry, R.J. (1981). Pretibial rash in *Legionella pneumophila* pneumonia. *JAMA* **245**, 1758–9.

Helms, C.M., Viner, J.P., Weisenburger, D.D., *et al.* (1984). Sporadic Legionnaires' disease. Clinical observations on 87 nosocomial and community acquired cases. *Am J Med Science* **288**, 2–12.

Herwaldt, L.A., Gorman, G.W., McGrath, T., *et al.* A new legionella species, *Legionella feeleii* species nova, causes Pontiac fever in an automobile plant. *Ann Intern Med* **100**, 333–8.

Holliday, P.L., Cullis, P.A. and Gilroy, J. (1982). Motor neuropathy in a patient with Legionnaires' disease. *Ann of Neurol* **12**, 493–4.

Holt, P. (1981). Legionnaires' disease and abscess of appendix. *Br Med J* **282**, 1035–6.

Huebner, R.E., Reeser, P.W. and Smith, D.W. (1984). Comparison of the virulence of the Philadelphia and Pontiac isolates of *Legionella pneumophila*. In *Legionella*: *Proceedings of the 2nd International Symposium, Washington, DC.*, pp. 123–4. Edited by Thornsberry, C., Balows, A., Feeley, J.C. and Jakubowski, W. American Society for Microbiology, Washington.

Hughes, J.A. and Anderson, P.B. (1985). Pulmonary cavitation, fibrosis and Legionnaires' disease. *Eur J Respir Dis* **66**, 59–61.

Humayun, H.M., Bird, T.J., Daugirdas, J.T., *et al.* (1981). Legionnaires' disease bacillus in bone marrow. *Can Med Assocn J* **125**, 1084–5.

Jenkins, P., Miller, A.C., Osman, J. *et al.* 1979). Legionnaires' disease: a clinical description of thirteen cases. *Br J Dis Chest*, **73**, 31–8.

Johnson, D.A. and Etter, H.S. (1984). Legionnaires' disease with rhabdomyolysis and acute reversible myoglobinuric renal failure. *Sthn Med J* **77**, 777–9.

Johnson, J.D., Raff, M.J. and Van Arsdall, J.A. (1984). Neurologic manifestations of Legionnaires' disease. *Medicine (Baltimore)* **63**, 303–10.

Joly, J.R. and Winn, W.C. (1984). Correlation of subtypes of *Legionella pneumophilia* defined by monoclonal antibodies with epidemiological classification of cases and environmental sources. *J Infect Dis* **150**, 667–71.

Kalweit, W.H., Winn, W.C., Rocco, T.A. and Girod, J.C.(1982). Haemodialysis fistula infections caused by *Legionella pneumophila*. *Ann Inter Med* **96**, 173–5.

Kennedy, D.H., Bone, I. and Weir, A.I. (1981). Early diagnosis of Legionnaires' disease: distinctive neurological findings. *Lancet* 1, 940–41.

Kerr, D.S., Brewis, R.A.L. and Macrae, A.D. (1978). Legionnaires' disease and acute renal failure. *Br Med J* 2, 538–9.

Kirby, B.D., Peck, H. and Meyer, R.D. (1979). Radiographic features of Legionnaires' disease. *Chest* 76, 562–5.

Kirby, B.D., Snyder, K.M., Meyer, R.D., and Finegold, S.M. (1980). Legionnaires' disease: Report of 65 nosocomial acquired cases and review of the literature. *Medicine* 59, 188–205.

Kovatch, A.L., Jardine, D.S., Dowling, J.N. *et al.* (1984). Legionellosis in children with leukaemia and relapse. *Paediatrics* 73, 811–15.

Kuritsky, J.N., Reingold, A.L., Hightower, A.W. and Broome, C.V. (1984). Sporadic legionellosis in the United States, 1970–1982. In *Legionella*: *Proceedings of the 2nd international Symposium, Washington, DC.*, pp. 243–5. Edited by Thornsberry, C., Balows, A., Feeley, J.C. and Jakubowski, W. American Society for Microbiology, Washington.

Landes, B.W., Pogson, G.W., Beauchamp, G.D., *et al.* (1982). Pericarditis in a patient with Legionnaires' disease. *Arch Intern Med*, 142, 1234–5.

Lattimer, G.L., Rhodes, L.V., Salventi, J.S. *et al.* (1979). The Philadelphia epidemic of Legionnaires' disease: clinical, pulmonary and serological findings two years later. *Ann Intern Med* 90, 522–6.

Lode, H., Schafer, H. and Ruckdeschel, G. (1982). Legionnaires' disease: prospective study of its incidence, clinical features and prognosis. *Duetsche Medizinische Wochenschrift* 107, 326–31.

Loveridge, P. (1981). Legionnaires' disease and arthritis. *Can Med Assocn J* 124, 366–7.

McCabe, R.E., Baldwin, J.C., McGregor, A., *et al.* (1984). Prosthetic valve endocarditis caused by *Legionella pneumophila*. *Ann Intern Med* 100, 525–7.

Macfarlane, J.T. (1983). Legionnaires' disease. *Practitioner* 227, 1707–18.

Macfarlane, J.T. and Macrae, A.D. (1983). Psittacosis. *Br Med Bull* 39, 163–7.

Macfarlane, J.T. and Neale, I.A. (1979). Rapid diagnosis of *Mycoplasma pneumoniae* infection: a reminder. *Br Med J* 1, 124.

Macfarlane, J.T. and Ward, M.J. (1982). Hyponatraemia in Legionnaires' disease. *Br Med J* 284, 1047.

Macfarlane, J.T., Miller, A.C., Roderick-Smith, W.H., *et al.* (1984). Comparative radiographic features of community acquired Legionnaires' disease, pneumococcal pneumonia, mycoplasma pneumonia and psittacosis. *Thorax* 39, 28–33.

Macfarlane, J.T., Ward, M.J., Finch, R.G. and Macrae, A.D. (1982). Hospital study of adult community-acquired pneumonia. *Lancet* 2, 255–8.

Macfarlane, J.T., Ward, M.J. and Mayhew, J. (1982). Creatine kinase and confusion in pneumonia. *Lancet* 2, 1221.

Macrae, A.D., Greaves, P.W. and Platts, P. (1979). Isolation of *Legionella pneumophila* from blood culture. *Br Med J* 2, 1189–90.

Marrie, T.J., Haldane, E.V., Noble, M.A. *et al.* (1981). Causes of atypical pneumonia: results of a one year prospective study. *Can Med Assocn J* 125, 118–23.

Marthedal, N.J. and Fisch-Thomsen, J. (1981). Legionnaires' disease with Guillain-Barre's syndrome. *Ugeskrift for Laeger* 143, 625.

Martin, R.S., Marrie, T.J., Best, L., *et al.* (1984). Isolation of *Legionella pneumophila* from the blood of a patient with Legionnaires' disease. *Can Med Assocn J* 131, 1085–7.

Maskill, M.R. and Jordan, E.C. (1981). Pronounced cerebellar features in Legionnaires' disease. *Br Med J* 283, 276.

Mayaud, C., Carette, M.F., Dournon, E., *et al.* (1984). Clinical features and prognosis of severe pneumonia caused by *Legionella pneumophila*. In *Legionella*:

Proceedings of the 2nd International Symposium, Washington, DC., pp. 11–12. Edited by Thornsberry, C., Balows, A., Feeley, J.C., and Jakubowski, W. American Society for Microbiology, Washington.

Maycock, R., Skale, B. and Kohler, I. (1983). *Legionella pneumophila* pericarditis proved by culture of pericardial fluid. *Am J Med* **75**, 534–6.

Milder, J.E. and Rough, R.R. (1982). Concurrent Legionnaires' disease and active pulmonary tuberculosis. *Am Rev Respir Dis* **125**, 759–61.

Miller, A.C. (1982). Hyponatraemia in Legionnaires' disease. *Br Med J* **284**, 558–9.

Miller, A.C. and Smith, W.H.R. (1978). Legionnaires' disease and bronchoscopy. *Lancet* **2**, 570.

Millunchick, E.W., Floyd, J. and Blanks, J. (1981). Legionnaires' disease in an immunologically normal child. *Am J Dis Childhood* **135**, 1065–6.

Mitchell, R.G., Pasvol, G. and Newnham, R.S. (1984). Pneumonia due to *Legionella bozemanii*: first report of a case in Europe. *J Infect* **8**, 251–5.

Morgan, D.J. and Gawler, J. (1981). Severe peripheral neuropathy complicating Legionnaires' disease. *Br Med J* **283**, 1577–8.

Muder, R.R., Reddy, S.C., Yu, V.L. and Kroboth, F.J. (1984). Pneumonia caused by Pittsburgh pneumonia agent: radiological manifestations. *Radiology* **150**, 633–7.

Muder, R.R., Yu, V.L., Vickers, R.M., *et al.* (1983). Simultaneous infection with *Legionella pneumophila* and Pittsburgh pneumonia agent. Clinical features and epidemiological implication. *Am J Med* **74**, 609–14.

Muder, R.R., Yu, V.L. and Zuravleff, J.J. (1983). Pneumonia due to Pittsburgh pneumonia agent: new clinical perspective with a review of the literature. *Medicine (Baltimore)* **62**, 120–8.

Nelson, D.P., Rensimer, E.R., Burke, C.M. and Raffin, T.A. (1984). Cardiac legionellosis (editorial). *Chest* **86**, 807–8.

Nelson, D.P., Rensimer, E.R. and Raffin, T.A. (1985). *Legionella pneumophila* pericarditis without pnenumonia. *Arch Intern Med* **145**, 926.

Nigro, G., Pastoris, M.C., Fantasia, M.M. and Midulla, M. (1983). Acute cerebellar ataxia in paediatric legionellosis. *Paediatrics* **72**, 847–9.

Oredugba, O., Mazumdar, D.C., Smoller, M.B., *et al.* (1980). Acute renal failure in Legionnaires' disease: report of a case. *Clin Nephrol* **13**, 142–5.

Orenstein, W.A., Overturf, G.D., Leedom, J.M., *et al.* (1981). The frequency of legionella infection prospectively determined in children hospitalized with pneumonia. *J Pediatr* **99**, 403–6.

Pastoris, M.C., Nigro, G., Mazzotti, M.F. and Midulla, M. (1984). *Legionella pneumophila* infection associated with arrhythmias and myocarditis in children without pneumonia. In *Legionella*: *Proceedings of the 2nd International Symposium, Washington, DC.*, pp. 14–15. Edited by Thornsberry, C., Balows, A., Feeley, J.C. and Jakubowski, W. American Society for Microbiology, Washington.

Pastoris, M.C., Nigro, G. and Midulla, M. (1985). Arrhythmia or myocarditis: a novel clinical form of *Legionella pneumophila* infection in children without pneumonia *Eur J Pediatr.* **144**, 157–9

Pearson, S.B. and Dadds, J.H.(1981). Neurological complication of Legionnaires' disease. *Postgrad Med J* **57**, 109–10.

Posner, M.R., Caudill, M.A., Brass, R. and Ellis, E. (1980). Legionnaires' disease associated with rhabdomyolysis and myoglobinurea. *Arch Intern Med* **140**, 848–50.

Poulter, N., Gabriel, R., Porter, K.A. *et al.* (1981). Acute interstitial nephritis complicating Legionnaires' disease. *Clin Nephrol* **15**, 216–20.

Renner, E.D., Helms, C.M., Hierholzer, W.J., *et al.* (1979). Legionnaires' disease in pneumonia patients in Iowa. A retrospective seroepidemiologic study. 1972–1979. *Ann Intern Med* **90**, 603–6.

Riggs, S.A., Wray, N.P., Waddell, C.C., *et al.* (1982). Thrombotic thrombocytopaenic purpura complicating Legionnaires' disease. *Arch Intern Med* **142**, 2275-80.

Rudin, J.E., Wing, E.J. and Yee, R.B. (1984). An ongoing outbreak of *Legionella micdadei*. In *Legionella: Proceedings of the 2nd International Symposium, Washington, DC.,* pp. 227-9. Edited by Thornsberry, C., Balows, A., Feeley, J.C. and Jakubowski, W. American Society for Microbiology, Washington.

Ryan, M.E., Feldman, S., Pruitt, B. and Fraser, D.W. (1979). Legionnaires' disease in a child with cancer. *Pediatrics* **64**, 951-3.

Saleh, F., Rodichok, L.D., Satya-Murti, S. and Tillotson, J.R. (1980). Legionnaires' disease. Report of a case with unusual manifestations. *Arch Intern Med* **140**, 1514-16.

Sato, P., Madtes, D.K., Thorning, D. and Albert, R.K. (1985). Bronchiolitis obliterans caused by *Legionella pneumophila*. *Chest* **87**, 840-2.

Schlanger, G., Lutwick, L.I., Kurzman, M., *et al.* (1984). Sinusitis caused by *Legionella pneumophila* in a patient with the acquired immune deficiency syndrome. *Am J Med* **77**, 957-60.

Simpson, R.M., Cogswell, J.J., Mitchell, E.R. and Macrae, A.D. (1980). Legionnaires' disease in an infant. *Lancet* **2**, 740-41.

Stamenkovic, I., Kurt, A.M., Montani, J.P. and Kapanci, Y. (1983). *Legionella dumoffii* pneumonia with adult respiratory distress syndrome. *Schweizerische Medizinische Wochenschrift* **113**, 608-12.

Strikas, R., Selfert, M.R. and Lentino, J.R. (1983). Autoimmune haemolytic anaemia and *Legionella pneumophila* pneumonia. *Ann Intern Med* **99**, 345.

Tsai, T.F., Finn, D.R., Plikaytis, B.D., *et al.* (1979) Legionnaires' disease: Clinical features of an epidemic in Philadelphia. *Ann Intern Med* **90**, 509-17.

Walder, M., Svanteson, B., Ursing, J., *et al.* (1981). Incidence of legionella pneumonia in acute lower respiratory tract infections. *Scan J Infec Dis* **13**, 159-60.

Watts, J.C., Hicklin, M.D., Thomason, B.M., *et al.* (1980). Fatal pneumonia caused by *Legionella pneumophila*, Serogroup 3: Demonstration of the bacilli in extra-thoracic organs. *Ann Intern Med* **92**, 186-8.

Wegmuller, E., Weidmann, P., Hess, T. and Reubi, F.C. (1985). Rapidly progressive glomerulonephritis accompaning Legionnaires' disease. *Arch Intern Med* **145**, 1711-13.

Weisenburger, D.D., Helms, C.M. and Renner, E.D. (1981). Sporadic Legionnaires' disease. *Arch Pathol Labor Med* **105**, 130-37.

White, R.J., Blainey, A.D., Harrison, K.J. and Clarke, S.K.R. (1981). Causes of pneumonia presenting to a district general hospital. *Thorax* **36**, 566-70.

Williams, M.E. Watanakunakorn, C., Baird, I.M. and Gerald, S.E. (1980). Legionnaires' disease with acute renal failure. *Am J Med Sc* **279**, 177-83.

Woodhead, M.A. and Macfarlane, J.T. (1985). The protean manifestations of Legionnaires' disease. *J R Coll Phys London* **19**, 224-30.

Woodhead, M.A. and Macfarlane, J.T. (1986a). Legionnaires' disease: a review of 79 community acquired cases in Nottingham. *Thorax* **41**, 635-40.

Woodhead, M.A. and Macfarlane, J.T. (1986b). Comparative features of legionella pneumonia with those of pneumococcal and mycoplasma pneumonia. *Br J Dis Chest* (in press).

Woodhead, M.A., Macfarlane, J.T., Macrae, A.D., and Pugh, S.F. (1986). The rise and fall of Legionnaires' disease in Nottingham. *J Infect* (in press).

Yu, V.L., Kroboth, F.J., Shonnard, J., *et al.* (1982). Legionnaires' disease: New clinical perspective from a prospective pneumonia study. *Am J Med* **73**, 357-61.

4 Management of Legionella Pneumonia

Two aspects of the management of legionella pneumonia will be discussed in this chapter. Firstly the management of a patient known to have legionella pneumonia will be considered. This will include both antibiotic therapy and also general supportive measures. Secondly, there is the patient who presents with either a community acquired pneumonia or a nosocomial pneumonia of unknown cause, in which legionella infection is one of the possibilities. This latter approach is important because usually the cause of the pneumonia is not known when a patient first presents and initial antibiotic therapy must be guided by a 'best guess' choice.

Management of a patient known to have legionella pneumonia

This is divided into antibiotic therapy and the equally important general supportive therapies.

Antibiotic therapy

Experimental evidence

Assessment of antibiotic therapy for legionella infections is still hampered by the lack of proper clinical trials, although there is a wealth of information from *in vitro* and animal studies. *L. pneumophila* is susceptible to a number of antibiotics *in vitro*. These include rifampicin, erythromycin, aminoglycosides, doxycycline, cefoxitin, chloramphenicol, beta-lactam antibiotics and co-trimoxazole (Saravolatz *et al.*, 1980; Thornsberry *et al.*, 1978; Weisholtz and Tomasz, 1985). In general, rifampicin is the most active agent against the different strains, with a minimum inhibitory concentration (MIC) of about 0.03 mg/ml, followed by erythromycin (MIC of about 0.2 mg/ml) (Ristuccia *et al.*, 1984). Of the tetracyclines, doxycycline appears to be the most active, followed by minocyclin. Various legionella species have been shown to produce beta-lactamase and other enzymes capable of hydrolysing beta-lactam substrates, and the activity of ampicillin and amoxycillin *in vitro* can be enhanced when combined with a beta-lactamase inhibitor such as clavulanate (Jones *et al.*, 1984). When the effect of ampicillin on the morphology and regrowth ability of *L. pneumophila* in broth culture is compared with that of erythromycin in the scanning electron microscope, the former (being bactericidal) delays regrowth to a greater extent than erythromycin (Rodgers and Elliott, 1984).

However, these *in vitro* studies have little relevance to the treatment of human infection as, *in vivo*, the legionella bacterium is an intracellular pathogen. In the lung the bacteria are phagocytosed by polymorphonuclear neutrophils and pulmonary macrophages. Many of the bacteria survive and can multiply in the macrophages, eventually disrupting the cell. Many bacteria are released to repeat the cycle (Baskerville, 1984). The ability of antibiotics to penetrate these pulmonary cells appears to be the major criterion for their efficacy. Rifampicin, and to a lesser extent erythromycin, are most effective at this. The situation is further complicated because electron microscopy reveals that the bacteria lie within membrane-bound vacuoles, in the cell cytoplasm (Horwitz and Silverstein, 1983). When rifampicin or erythromycin is added to cultured human blood monocytes, infected with *L. pneumophila*, the intracellular multiplication of the bacteria is inhibited but they are not killed. This inhibition is reversible after the antibiotic is removed from the tissue culture.

In studies of the ability of various antibiotics to prevent death of embryonated hens' eggs infected with *L. pneumophila*, only rifampicin and erythromycin give complete protection against death of the embryo (Lewis *et al.*, 1978). Similar results have been found with animal models. Of guinea-pigs infected by intraperitoneal injection of *L. pneumophila* only those treated with rifampicin or erythromycin survived (Fraser *et al.*, 1978). Of the tetracyclines, only doxycycline significantly prolonged survival of infected animals (Yoshida *et al.*, 1985). However, the illness in these animal models cannot be compared directly with human disease because infection was not caused by inhalation of the organisms.

More clinically relevant animal experiments have come from exposing guinea-pigs and monkeys to aerosol suspensions of broth cultures of *L. pneumophila* and studying the pathological and bacteriological effects after different antibiotics (Gibson *et al.*, 1983). A comparison was made between the efficacy of erythromycin, gentamicin and rifampicin, given in doses similar to, or up to 4 times the typical human dose, adjusted by weight. All three antibiotics prevented death after a minimal (1 × LD50) infection but rifampicin was the only antibiotic to prevent death after a 10 × LD50 infecting dose. Rifampicin was also the most effective antibiotic in preventing the progression of the pneumonia histologically and by the clearance of *L. pneumophila* from the lungs. The results for gentamicin were superior to those of erythromycin.

Clinical experience

There have been no clinical trials with different antibiotics for legionella pneumonia in man and we have to rely on experience from several uncontrolled clinical studies for information about the effectiveness of various antibiotics. As many patients with severe pneumonia may have received several different antibiotics, assessment of the relative efficacy of each is difficult. The overall impression from case fatality studies is that

Table 4.1 Mortality and antibiotic treatment for legionella pneumonia from published series. Many patients were treated with more than one antibiotic and death and survival has been assigned to all drugs received. (Broome *et al.*, 1979**; Bouza *et al.*, 1984; Carter, J.B., 1979; Gump *et al.*, 1979; Helms *et al.*, 1984**; Kennedy and Borland, 1983*; Kirby *et al.*, 1980; Marrie *et al.*, 1981; Meenhorst *et al.*, 1979; Nordstrom *et al.*, 1983; Saravolatz *et al.*, 1979; Tsai *et al.*, 1979; Woodhead and Macfarlane, 1986)

	Mortality	No. deaths/No. treated
Erythromycin	9.6 %	29/301
Tetracycline	5 %	3/60
Ampicillin	22 %	26/117
Other penicillins	28 %	39/140
Cephalosporins	32 %	41/130
Chloramphenicol	31 %	5/16
Aminoglycosides	34 %	36/106

*   Data not complete
** Study shows statistically significant reduction in mortality with erythromycin

erythromycin therapy is associated with the lowest mortality and it is, at present, the recommended antibiotic therapy for legionella pneumonia. Patients with a mild infection can be treated orally but those who are moderately or severely ill require intravenous therapy (Table 4.1). Generally patients cannot tolerate oral doses of erythromycin greater than 2 g daily because of gastro-intestinal side-effects. Phlebitis at the cannula site has occurred in up to half the patients given intravenous erythromycin (Macfarlane *et al.*, 1983) but this problem can be partially overcome by a slow, dilute infusion. It is generally recommended that treatment should continue for at least 3 weeks because relapse or slow recovery has been reported in some patients treated for shorter periods (Kirby *et al.*, 1980). However, this may not be necessary in patients with mild disease and indeed patients do recover without ever having received erythromycin therapy. Thus factors other than antibiotic treatment may also influence the course of the disease (Helms *et al.*, 1984).

Experimental data strongly supports the efficacy of rifampicin in the treatment of legionella infection but reported clinical experience is limited. However, use of rifampicin, together with erythromycin, is recommended in patients with legionella pneumonia who are critically ill or severely immuno-suppressed or who have lung abscesses. Rifampicin should not be given alone because of the potential development of resistance. Where erythromycin cannot be given for any reason, then the lipid-soluble tetracycline, doxy-cycline, could be used alone or with rifampicin. Reports suggest that this may be effective although again experience is limited (Table 4.2).

Of the newer antibiotics, the quinolones look promising. Ciprofloxacin appears to be particularly effective when given both parenterally and by the aerosol route to guinea-pigs infected by inhalation of *L. pneumophila*. (Fitzgeorge *et al.*, 1985; Fitzgeorge, *et al.*, 1986). It was as effective as rifampicin and considerably better than erythromycin in reducing the number of bacteria in the lung and preventing death (Fitzgeorge *et al.*, 1986). Being very lipid soluble, it penetrates macrophages well. Reported clinical experience with ciprofloxacin is limited (Winter *et al.*, 1986).

Table 4.2 Recommended antibiotic therapy for a patient with proven or suspected legionella pneumonia (adapted from Edelstein, 1984)

	Drug	Route	Daily dose adults
Mild illness	i. Erythromycin	Oral	500 mg, 6 hourly
	ii. Doxycycline (?)	Oral	200 mg STAT and 100 mg, 12 hourly
Moderate or severe illness	i. Erythromycin	IV*	1 g, 6 hourly
	ii. Add Rifampicin	IV, oral	600 mg, 12 hourly
	iii. Doxycycline (?)	IV	200 mg STAT and 100 mg, 12 hourly

* Intravenous
Rifampicin should not be given alone. Clinical experience with doxycycline is limited

Antibiotic therapy for other legionella species
L. micdadei and the other legionella species are sensitive *in vitro* to a wide variety of antibiotics (Dowling *et al.*, 1982; Jones *et al.*, 1984). *L. micdadei* is relatively more sensitive to beta-lactam drugs *in vitro* than *L. pneumophila*. This is partially due to the absence of a beta-lactamase (Jones *et al.*, 1984). However, only erythromycin, rifampicin and co-trimoxazole protect guinea-pigs from fatal infections with *L. micdadei* (Muder *et al.*, 1983). Although there are case reports of successful treatment with co-trimoxazole (Rudin *et al.*, 1984) and ampicillin (Macfarlane *et al.*, 1981), erythromycin (together with rifampicin in severe infection) is regarded as the therapy of choice for *L. micdadei* and the other legionella species (Muder *et al.*, 1983).

General supportive measures

The general management of the patient with moderate or severe pneumonia is very important and is often done badly. Fever and pleural pain can usually be relieved by regular aspirin or indomethacin. Patients can be dehydrated or hypovolaemic and adequate hydration is essential either by the oral or intravenous route. For patients with moderate or severe pneumonia significant hypoxia is common and its correction very important. They should receive enough added oxygen through an appropriate oxygen mask to bring the arterial oxygen up to a safe level. An arterial oxygen concentration of 6.6 Kpa (50 mmHg) or less, a rising arterial carbon dioxide and acidosis indicate severe pneumonia and respiratory failure. Assisted ventilation may well be required. This can be life-saving and should be started early.

Patients with severe pneumonia are best managed on an intensive therapy unit or similar high dependency area where they can be carefully monitored and their arterial blood gases checked frequently. Sudden death occurring in such patients managed on general medical wards, may often be due to unsuspected and therefore inadequately treated hypoxia, and acute respiratory failure (Woodhead *et al.*, 1985). In patients with legionella pneumonia who require assisted ventilation for respiratory failure the outlook is not hopeless and the recovery rate can be over 50 per cent (Woodhead and Macfarlane, 1986). Vigorous chest physiotherapy and postural drainage is not usually helpful in the acute stage of a pneumonia and may merely serve to exhaust a toxic and ill patient.

Patients who are confused are a particular management problem especially when they are intolerant of oxygen therapy by mask. On occasions, assisted ventilation is required for a period to allow adequate sedation at the same time as correcting hypoxia. Adequate nutrition during the acute illness is essential and nutritional support should be started if protein calorie intake has been insufficient for 48 hours or longer. Enteral (by nasogastric tube) or parenteral feeding may be needed for patients unable to maintain adequate oral nutrition.

Prognosis

The two most important factors affecting outcome include the state of the patients' health before the infection and the therapy given for the infection. The relationship between antibiotics and fatality rates has already been discussed. The mortality rate in previously healthy individuals is low, in the order of 5–15 per cent. In contrast the mortality in patients who are immunosuppressed can approach 70–80 per cent.

Management of the patient presenting with community acquired pneumonia

Recent studies have helped to clarify the relative importance of different pathogens causing community acquired pneumonia in adults (British Thoracic Society Research Committee, 1986; Macfarlane *et al.*, 1982; McNabb *et al.*, 1984; White *et al.*, 1981). The main conclusion is that community acquired pneumonia is caused by a limited number of pathogens. Pneumococcal infection is the commonest and is implicated in up to a half or three-quarters of cases. Other bacterial infections are really quite uncommon and in particular Gram-negative infections are very unusual. Staphyloccocal pneumonia is rare except during an influenza virus epidemic. The reported incidence of legionella pneumonia varies, depending on where, when and how it is looked for. Viral infections and atypical pneumonias caused by *M. pneumoniae, Coxiella burnetii* and *Chlamydia psittaci* may on occasions form a sizeable group. Such considerations have important implications for deciding on antibiotic treatment when the patient is first seen.

Investigating the cause of community acquired pneumonia

If the patient is ill enough to require hospital admission, it is important to try and identify the cause of the pneumonia as soon as possible. Sputum, blood and, if available, pleural fluid should be collected for Gram staining and culture before antibiotics are started. Even a single dose of antibiotic may impede the growth of common pathogens such as *S. pneumoniae* or *H. influenzae*. Sometimes sputum culture may be misleading because of contamination of the lower respiratory tract secretions as they pass through the oropharynx. In addition, a first blood sample should be collected early in the illness for testing antibody titres to viruses, atypical pathogens and legionella species. Serological tests should be repeated 10–14 days later or during convalescence to look for a rising antibody titre.

Only a proportion of microbiology laboratories in the United Kingdom can provide a routine serological service for legionella diagnosis and sera are sent to a reference laboratory. A close liaison is therefore essential between the clinician and the microbiologist to ensure appropriate and rapid investigations.

If the patient is seriously ill or fails to improve, invasive techniques should be considered to obtain lower respiratory tract secretions if initial tests have failed to find a cause for the pneumonia. These techniques include transtracheal aspiration, percutaneous lung aspiration and fibreoptic bronchoscopy to obtain samples of bronchial secretions, bronchoalveolar lavage fluid and transbronchial lung biopsies from specified areas of the lung (Chiodini *et al.*, 1985; Macfarlane, 1985). Bronchial aspirates were particularly useful in making an early diagnosis of legionella pneumonia in one study (Winter *et al.*, 1986).

Antibiotic choice for community acquired pneumonia

The cause of the pneumonia is not usually known when the patient is first seen and in practice a 'best guess' antibiotic choice has to be made. This will depend on the patient, the severity of infection and any aetiological clues from the clinical picture. Most patients with mild pneumonia, treated at home or in hospital, respond rapidly to antibiotics such as amoxycillin, erythromycin or co-trimoxazole. Patients with more severe pneumonia need to be identified early because deterioration may be rapid and mortality is significant even in previously fit people. As soon as specimens have been taken for bacterial culture, antibiotic therapy should be started.

Because pneumococcal infection is still the commonest cause of community acquired pneumonia the antibiotic chosen must provide effective cover against it. Other likely causes of severe community acquired pneumonia include legionella infection, psittacosis, Q fever, and mycoplasma pneumonia. High doses of intravenous penicillin (4–8 megaU daily) and erythromycin (2–4 g daily) given together provide good initial cover for these pathogens. Ampicillin (2–4 g daily) should replace penicillin in patients who have chronic lung disease, such as chronic bronchitis, where infection by *H. influenzae* is more likely. Patients who are allergic to penicillins can be given erythromycin alone in high doses. Staphylococcal pneumonia is uncommon except during an epidemic of influenza virus during the winter. At such times, or if staphylococcal pneumonia is suspected, flucloxacillin or another antistaphylococcal agent should be used as well. The antibiotics are adjusted appropriately if cultures or other investigations identify a specific pathogen. When routine cultures of blood, sputum and other body fluids are negative in a patient with severe pneumonia, the likelihood of a legionella infection should be reconsidered and thought given to adding rifampicin therapy if the patient is deteriorating.

In one study of adults admitted to an intensive care unit with community acquired pneumonia, half of the patients in whom a diagnosis had not been made by routine bacteriological techniques by 48 hours, were subsequently found to have legionella pneumonia (Woodhead *et al.*, 1985).

Management of the patient with a nosocomial pneumonia

The management of a patient with a nosocomial pneumonia of unknown cause is more complex (Santoro, 1984). Nosocomial pneumonia usually arises from aspiration of nasopharyngeal contents, inhalation of bacteria from contaminated equipment or, rarely, by blood spread from a distant infected site (as may occur with abdominal sepsis). Colonization of the nasopharynx with Gram-negative bacteria occurs rapidly in half of the patients who enter hospital. Illness, impaired consciousness and any neurological disease will make aspiration of such pathogens more likely. Immunosuppression, either from underlying disease or from drug therapy, reduces local pulmonary defences. General anaesthetics, thoracic and abdominal surgery and reduced cough reflex impair clearance of pathogens from the bronchopulmonary tree. Inhalation of pathogenic bacteria from contaminated respiratory equipment in areas, such as intensive care units, exacerbate the problem. Many outbreaks of nosocomial legionella pneumonia have also been caused by colonization of hospital heating, ventilation and water systems.

The spectrum of pathogens encountered in nosocomial pneumonia is much wider and more varied than for community acquired pneumonia. Gram-negative organisms comprise over half of all isolates and of the Gram-positive bacteria implicated, *S. aureus* is the commonest. In hospitals where it is endemic or epidemic, legionella infection can cause a significant number of cases. The potential list of pathogens causing nosocomial pneumonia in patients who are immunocompromised is even more varied and includes protozoal infection by *Pneumocystis carinii* and fungal infections caused by Aspergillus and Candida.

Every effort should be made to make an early aetiological diagnosis. Invasive techniques to obtain lung secretions should be considered at an early stage in these patients, if initial microbiological and serological tests are unhelpful. Fibreoptic bronchoscopy is probably the most rewarding and safe procedure. Specimens can be obtained of bronchial secretions, bronchoalveolar lavage fluid and transbronchial lung biopsies (Macfarlane, 1985). The technique of bronchoalveolar lavage is particularly helpful for diagnosing opportunistic infection (Hopkin *et al.*, 1983). In patients who are deteriorating rapidly an open lung biopsy should be considered (Gaensler, 1981). The ability to diagnose the cause of the pneumonia from an open lung biopsy in the immunocompromised patient is high and the morbidity and mortality relatively low, even in the seriously ill (Macfarlane, 1985; Venn *et al.*, 1985; Young, 1984).

Antibiotic therapy for a patient with nosocomial pneumonia

Because of the wide variety of potential pathogens, a broad spectrum antibiotic or a combination of antibiotics is needed as initial therapy, pending the results of bacteriological and serological tests (Donowitz and Mandell, 1983). There are several antibiotics that would be suitable but a good choice would be a broad spectrum third generation cephalosporin (or penicillin derivative such as ticarcillin, azlocillin or piperacillin), with or without an amino-glycoside, such as gentamicin. In institutions where legionella infection is a possibility, erythromycin therapy should also be considered.

Prevention of legionella pneumonia

Person-to-person transmission of legionella infection has not been convincingly documented. Therefore expensive and inconvenient barrier nursing' and special precautions for patients in hospital with legionella pneumonia are not required, and are impractical during a large epidemic (Rashed *et al.*, 1986). It would seem sensible, however, to dispose of respiratory secretions in the routine manner employed for other potentially infectious material, during the early stage of the illness (Jarvis, 1982). In patients acquiring a nosocomial infection the source of the infection should be investigated as outlined in Chapter 8. In sporadic cases it is rarely possible to identify a source but clustering of cases indicates the need for an epidemiological investigation.

Chemoprophylaxis has been suggested as a means of protecting immuno-suppressed patients at risk of legionella pneumonia, but experience is limited (Van Furth, 1984). In a transplantation unit in Belgium, 12 of 26 episodes of pneumonia were found to be due to legionella infection. Oral erythromycin (1.5–3 g per day) was subsequently given to patients during 39 episodes of high dose immunosuppression whilst eradication of the organism from the water supply was completed. No cases of legionella pneumonia occurred in this group in contrast to five cases in nine other severely immunosuppressed patients who did not receive chemoprophylaxis (Vereerstraeten *et al.*, 1986). Although much experimental work has been done on the immune responses to legionella infections, no progress has been made in developing a vaccine in humans (Eisenstein *et al.*, 1984).

References

Baskerville, A. (1984). Pathology and pathophysiology. In *Legionella: Proceedings of the 2nd International Symposium, Washington, DC.*, pp. 36–41. Edited by Thornsberry, C., Balows, A., Feeley, J.C. and Jakubowski, W. American Society for Microbiology, Washington.

Bouza, E. and Rodriguez-Creixems, M. (1984). Legionnaires' disease in Spain. In *Legionella: Proceedings of the 2nd International Symposium, Washington, DC.*, pp. 15–17. Edited by Thornsberry, C., Balows, A., Feeley, J.C. and Jakubowski, W. American Society for Microbiology, Washington.

British Thoracic Society Research Committee. (1986). Community acquired pneumonia in adults in British Hospitals in 1982–1983: A BTS/PHLS survey of aetiology, mortality, prognostic factors and outcome. *QJM*. In press.

Brooms, C.V., Goings, S.A., Thacker, S.B. *et al.* (1979). The Vermont epidemic of Legionnaires' disease. *Ann Intern Med* **90**, 573–7.

Carter, J.B. (1979). Legionnaires' disease at a community hospital. *Ann Intern Med* **91**, 794.

Chiodini, P.L., Williams, A.J., Barker, J. and Innes, J.A. (1985). Bronchial lavage and transbronchial lung biopsy in the diagnosis of Legionnaires' disease. *Thorax* **40**, 154–5.

Davis, G.S., Winn, W.C. and Beaty, H.N. (1981). Legionnaires' disease. *Clin Chest Med* **2**, 145–66.

Donowitz, G.R. and Mandell, G.L. (1983). Empiric therapy for pneumonia. *Rev Infect Dis* **5**, 40–51.

Dowling, J.D., Weyant, R.S. and Pasculle, W.A. (1982). Bactericidal activity of antibiotics against *Legionella micdadei* (Pittsburgh pneumonia agent). *Antimicr Agents Chemother* **22**, 272–6.

Edelstein, P.H. and Meyer, R.D. (1984). Legionnaires' disease. A review. *Chest* **85**, 114–20.

Eisenstein, T.K., Tamada, R., Meissler, J. *et al.* (1984). Vaccination against *Legionella pneumophila. Infection and Immunity* **45**, 685–91.

Fitzgeorge, R.B., Baskerville, A. and Featherstone, A.S.R. (1986). Treatment of experimental Legionnaires' disease by aerosol administration of rifampicin, ciprofloxacin and erythromycin. *Lancet* **1**, 502–3.

Fitzgeorge, R.B., Gibson, D.H., Jepras, K.I. and Baskerville, A. (1985). Studies on ciprofloxacin therapy of experimental Legionnaires' disease. *J Infect* **10** 194–203.

Fraser, D.W., Wachsmuth, I.K., Bopp, C. *et al.* (1978). Antibiotic treatment of guinea pigs infected with agent of Legionnaires' disease. *Lancet* **1**, 175–8.

Gaensler, E.A. (1981). Open and Closed Lung Biopsy. In *Diagnostic Techniques in Pulmonary Disease Part II*, pp. 597–622. Edited by Sackner, M.A. Marcel Dekker Inc., New York.

Gibson, D.H., Fitzgeorge, R.B. and Baskerville, A. (1983). Antibiotic therapy of experimental airborne Legionnaires' disease. *J Infect* **7**, 210–17.

Gump, D.W., Frank, R.O., Winn, W.C. *et al.* (1979). Legionnaires' disease in patients with associated severe disease. *Ann Intern Med* **90**, 538–42.

Helms, C.M., Viner, J.P., Weisenburger, D.D. *et al.* (1984). Sporadic Legionnaires' disease. Clinical observations on 87 nosocomial and community acquired cases. *Am J Med Sc* **288**, 2–12.

Hopkin, J.M., Turney, J.H., Young, J.A. *et al.* (1983). Rapid diagnosis of obscure pneumonia in immunosuppressed renal patients by cytology of alveolar lavage fluid. *Lancet* **2**, 299–301.

Horwitz, M.A. and Silverstein, S.C. (1983). Intracellular multiplication of Legionnaires' disease bacteria (*Legionella pneumophila*) in human monocytes is reversibly inhibited by erythromycin and rifampicin. *J Clin Invest* **71**, 15–26.

Jarvis, W.R. (1982). Recommended precautions for patients with Legionnaires' disease. *Infect Cont* **3**, 401–2.

Jones, R.N., McDougal, L.K. and Thornsberry, C. (1984). Inhibition and hydrolysis studies of beta lactamases found in Legionella species: Antimicrobial activity of new macrolides on legionellae. In *Legionella: Proceedings of the 2nd International Symposium, Washington, DC.*, pp. 100–103. Edited by Thornsberry, C., Balows, A., Feeley, J.C. and Jakubowski, W. American Society for Microbiology, Washington.

Kennedy, D.H. and Borland, W. (1983). How common is Legionnaires' disease? *Lancet* **1**, 360–1.

Kirby, B.D., Synder, K.M., Meyer, R.D. and Finegold, S.M. (1980). Legionnaires' disease: Report of 65 nosocomially acquired cases and review of the literature. *Medicine* **59**, 188–205.

Lewis, V.J., Thacker, W.L., Sheppard, C.C. *et al.* (1978). *In vivo* susceptibility of Legionnaires' bacterium to ten antimicrobial agents. *Antimicr Agents Chemother* **13**, 419–22.

Macfarlane, J.T. (1985). Lung biopsy. *Br Med J* **290**, 97–8.

Macfarlane, J.T., Finch, R.G., Laverick, A. and Macrae, A.D. (1981). Pittsburgh pneumonia agent and legionellosis in Nottingham. *Br Med J* **283**, 1222.

Macfarlane, J.T., Finch, R.G., Ward, M.J. and Rose, D.H. (1983). Erythromycin compared with a combination of ampicillin and amoxycillin as initial therapy for adults with pneumonia including Legionnaires' disease. *J Infect* **7**, 111–17.

Macfarlane, J.T., Ward, M.J., Finch, R.G. and Macrae, A.D. (1982). Hospital study of adult community acquired pneumonia. *Lancet* **2**, 255–8.

Marrie, T.J., Haldane, E.V., Noble, M.A. *et al.* (1981). Causes of atypical pneumonia: results of a one year prospective study. *Can Med J* **125**, 118–23.

McNabb, W.R., Shanson, D.C., Williams, T.D.M. and Lant, A.F. (1984). Adult community acquired pneumonia in Central London. *J R Soc Med* **77**, 550–5.

Meenhost, P.L., van der Meer, J.W. and Borst, J. (1979). Sporadic cases of Legionnaires' disease in the Netherlands. *Ann Intern Med* **90**, 529–32.

Muder, R.R., Yu, V.L. and Zuravleff, J.J. (1983). Pneumonia due to Pittsburgh pneumonia agent: new clinical perspective with a review of the literature. *Medicine* **62**, 120–8.

Nordstrom, K., Kallings, I., Dahnsjo, H. and Clemens, F. (1983). An outbreak of Legionnaires' disease in Sweden: Report of sixty eight cases. *Scand J Infect Dis* **15**, 43–55.

Rashed, K., Gibson, J., Fairfax, A. *et al.* (1986). Legionnaires' disease in Stafford: Management of an epidemic. *Lancet* **1**, 197–9.

Ristuccia, P.A., Cunha, B.A. and Ristuccia, A.M. (1984). *In vitro* activity of antimicrobial agents against *Legionella pneumophila* and type strains of four other legionella species. In *Legionella: Proceedings of the 2nd International Symposium, Washington, DC.*, pp. 99–100. Edited by Thornsberry, C., Balows, A., Feeley, J.C. and Jakubowski, W. American Society for Microbiology, Washington.

Rodgers, F.G. and Elliott, T.S. (1984). Action of ampicillin and erythromycin on the growth and morphology of *Legionella pneumophila*. In *Legionella: Proceedings of the 2nd International Symposium, Washington, DC.*, pp. 103–5. Edited by Thornsberry, C., Balows, A., Feeley, J.C. and Jakubowski, W. American Society for Microbiology, Washington.

Rudin, J.E., Evans, T.L. and Wing, E.J. (1984). Failure of erythromycin in treatment of *Legionella micdadei* pneumonia. *Am J Med* **76**, 318–20.

Santoro, J. (1984). Nosocomial Respiratory Tract Infection. In *The Pneumonias*, pp. 182–96. Edited by Levison, M.E. Wright. PSG, Boston.

Saravolatz, L.D., Pohlod, D.J. and Quinn, E.L. (1980). Antimicrobial susceptibility of *Legionella pneumophila* serogroups I–IV. *Scand J Infec Dis* **12**, 215–19.

Thornsberry, C.L., Baker, C.N. and Kirven, L.A. (1978). *In vitro* activity of antimicrobial agents on Legionnaires' disease bacterium. *Antimicr Agents Chemother* **13**, 78–80.

Tsai, T.F., Finn, D.R., Plikaytis, B.D. (1979). Legionnaires' disease: Clinical features of an epidemic in Philadelphia. *Ann Intern Med* **90**, 509–17.

Van Furth, R. (1984). Some views on the immune responses in legionella infections. In *Legionella: Proceedings of the 2nd International Symposium, Washington, DC.*, pp. 199–201. Edited by Thornsberry, C., Balows, A., Feeley, J.C. and Jakubowski, W. American Society for Microbiology, Washington.

Vereerstraeten, P., Stolear, J.C., Schoutens-Serruys, E. *et al.* (1986). Erythromycin prophylaxis for Legionnaires' disease in immunosuppressed patients in a contaminated hospital environment. *Transplantation* **41**, 52–4.

Venn, G.E., Kay, P.H., Midwood, C.J. and Goldstraw, P. (1985). Open lung biopsy in patients with diffuse pulmonary shadowing. *Thorax* **40**, 931–5.

Weisholtz, S. and Tomas, Z.A. (1985). Response of *Legionella pneumophila to beta lactam antibiotics. Antimicr Agents Chemother* **27**, 695–700.

White, R.J., Blainey, A.D., Harrison, K.J. and Clarke, S.K.R. (1981). Causes of pneumonia presenting to a district general hospital. *Thorax* **36**, 566–70.

Winter, J.H., McCartney, A.C., Fallon, R.J. *et al.* (1986). Outbreak of Legionnaires' disease at Glasgow Royal Infirmary: early containment by rapid diagnosis. *Thorax.* Abstract, in press.

Woodhead, M.A. and Macfarlane, J.T. (1986). Legionnaires' disease: a review of 79 community acquired cases in Nottingham. *Thorax* **41**, 635–40.

Woodhead, M.A., Macfarlane, J.T., Rodgers, F.G. *et al.* (1985). Aetiology and outcome of severe community-acquired pneumonia. *J Infect* **10**, 204–10.

Yoshida, S., Mizuguchi, Y., Ohta, H. and Ogawa, M. (1985). Effects of tetracyclines on experimental *Legionella pneumophila* infection in guinea pigs. *J Antimicrob Chemoth* **16**, 199–204.

Young, L.S. (1984). *Pneumocystis Carinii Pneumonia*, pp. 156–74. Marcel Dekker Inc., New York.

5 Pathology

Legionnaires' disease first became evident as a severe, sometimes fatal pneumonia. Although this is still a dominant characteristic, the infection is now known to range from the mild non-specific illness known as Pontiac fever, without lung involvement, through to extensive consolidation affecting one or both lungs. Despite a variety of presenting symptoms, the pathological changes at autopsy, where the gross appearances resemble those of other severe respiratory infections, are confined almost entirely to lung tissue. However, dissemination of the causative organisms to other sites via lymphatic and haematogenous pathways has been described and these sites included hilar lymph nodes, spleen, kidneys, liver, bone marrow, brain and muscle including heart.

Deaths have occurred from shortly after onset almost up to the stage of resolution of the disease, with a mean survival time between 8 and 13 days.

Macroscopic appearance of lung

At death one or both lungs may appear swollen with the cyanosed picture of lobar consolidation. In some instances straw-coloured or sero-sanguinous fluid, variable in amount, is present in the pleural cavity; in others a fibrinous exudate binds the pleural surfaces together. The disease may develop in any lobe of either lung, though, once established, it is inclined to spread rapidly, particularly in those with underlying problems including immunologic deficiency. On removal, the affected lungs are airless and heavy, often weighing more than 1000 g.

Depending on the duration of illness, the cut surface of the lung shows focal or lobar consolidation (see Plate 1) with surrounding oedema and congestion and red or, more often, grey hepatization. Akin to infarction, the tissue may appear necrotic and particularly after fixation, can feel caseous and friable when scraped. Other findings have included small haemorrhagic areas or early focal abscess formation from release of bacterial toxins (Blackmon *et al.*, 1978; Boyd *et al.*, 1978; Winn and Myerowitz, 1981). Rarely as in dual infections of immunocompromised individuals multiple lung abscess and disseminated intravascular coagulation have been reported (Dowling *et al.*, 1983).

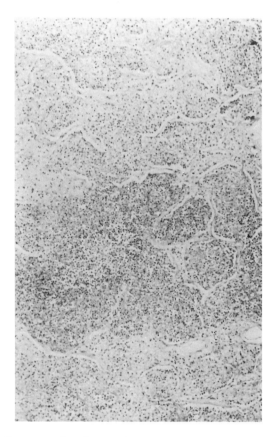

Fig. 5.1 Legionella pneumonia: microscopic appearance of severe inflammatory response in lung. (H and E section, low power.)

Microscopic appearance of lung

Affected lung tissue on section characteristically exhibits a severe inflammatory response indicative of acute fibrino-purulent pneumonia (Fig. 5.1). Alveoli and terminal bronchioles are distended with proteinaceous fibrin-rich debris in which macrophages and neutrophil polymorphonuclear leucocytes are present in varying numbers and proportions. These cells may show degenerative changes proceeding to areas of necrosis though the extent of this effect is governed by the severity of the illness and its duration before death. Among other features which may be observed are focal hyperplasia in alveoli with desquamation of lining cells, some interstitial oedema and infiltration with lymphocytes and neutrophils, low grade vasculitis with occasional thrombi, or small haemorrhages into alveolar spaces. Larger bronchioles are not usually damaged though they may be filled with exudate. When the lung is covered with a layer of fibrinous pleurisy this usually contains scanty numbers of lymphocytes. In reports from the United States (Blackmon *et al.*, 1978; Hicklin *et al.*, 1980) hyaline membrane formation has been noted in lung showing acute diffuse alveolar damage though other

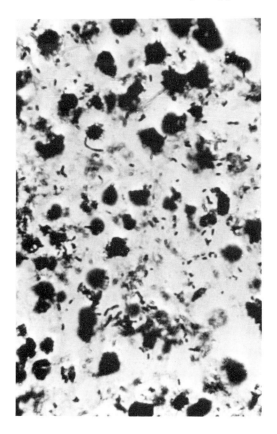

Fig. 5.2 Legionella pneumonia: microscopic appearance of lung with organisms stained by Warthin-Starry method (× 1000).

factors such as oxygen toxicity or shock may account for it at least in part. Hyaline membranes were not observed in material from Scottish cases (Boyd *et al.*, 1978). Immunosuppressed patients tend to react adversely when exposed to legionella infection, the fibrino-serous alveolar exudate showing a poor inflammatory response (Weisenburger *et al.*, 1981).

In legionella pneumonias the process of resolution even when death occurs at a late stage of the illness appears minimal. Among survivors this is corroborated by the slow clearance of lung shadowing, sometimes taking up to 3–5 months from onset. On occasion, it is accompanied by intrapulmonary streaky opacities indicative of healing associated with fibrosis (Macfarlane *et al.*, 1984). These alveolar and interstitial fibrotic changes result from organization of the fibrin and hyaline membrane and lead to obliteration of areas of lung with impairment of lung function. They cannot be distinguished from other types of pneumonia which fail to resolve (Blackmon *et al.*, 1979).

Currently, many legionella species have been shown to cause human pneumonia, though since its discovery in 1977 *L. pneumophila* serogroup 1 has remained the dominant organism. In keeping with a mode of infection arising from inhalation, these small Gram-negative rods may be found in lung tissue in considerable profusion during the early stage of the illness. Despite the slow progress in resolution already noted, their numbers, particularly in immunocompetent patients, decline steadily as the disease progresses and usually disappear from the lung tissue by the end of the second week. However among those immunocompromised and showing a poor inflammatory response the organisms may be found over a longer period.

In stained sections of lung the legionella organisms are not visualized by haematoxylin and eosin. Among other stains tried, the most successful, though it is not strictly specific, has been silver impregnation by the Dieterle or Warthin-Starry methods (Fig. 5.2). Specific identification has been possible by the fluorescence antibody technique either directly with fluorescein-conjugated antisera or indirectly by the use of a range of specific antisera which can then be overlayed by an appropriate anti-human or anti-animal globulin conjugate (see Plate 2). The great value of fluorescence is that it can be done on impression smears of freshly cut lung surface after acetone fixation, on smears of scrapings from fresh or formalin-fixed lung surfaces or on deparaffined formalin-fixed lung sections. With the use of a panel of monoclonal antibodies it is becoming practicable to identify the subgroup of strains in such tissues and even to pinpoint their source (Brown *et al.*, 1985).

Electron microscopy

Electron microscopy can also help to establish the identity of legionella species in affected lung tissue (Rodgers 1979, 1983). Both negative staining of extracts and examination of thin sections will indicate the presence of organisms with the appropriate size and morphological appearance. Confirmation of identity is then possible by a specific immunoferritin technique. In addition, it has shown the species to be facultative intracellular pathogens, invading and multiplying within lung macrophages. This can aid their survival by circumventing humoral immunity and, by their intracellular propagation, allow release of toxic products. It may also assist in explaining spread by blood to other parts of the body.

Other tissues

Legionella organisms or antigens, together with evidence of some inflammatory reaction have been demonstrated in several extrathoracic sites including myocardium (White *et al.*, 1980) spleen, bone marrow, kidneys (Weisenburger *et al.*, 1981), brain (Gatell *et al.*, 1981), peritoneum (Dournon *et al.*, 1982), pericardium (Maycock *et al.*, 1983; Nelson *et al.*, 1985), maxillary sinuses (Schlanger *et al.*, 1984) and in vegetations on mitral and aortic valve replacements (McCabe *et al.*, 1984). These findings are thought to result from bacteraemia, the associated pathological changes being minor and non-specific. Though the disease can give rise to confusion and other manifestations of cerebral disturbance (Bernardini *et al.*, 1985; Lees and

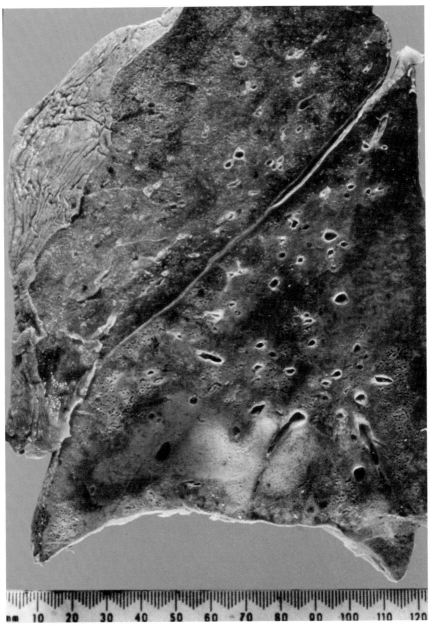

Plate 1 Legionella pneumonia: cut surface showing lobar consolidation. (Photograph kindly provided by Dr J.S.P. Jones.)

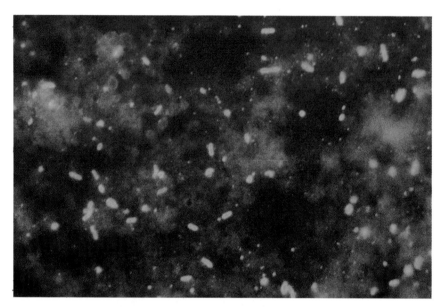

Plate 2 Legionella pneumonia: organisms in lung tissue, fluorescent antibody stain (× 1000).

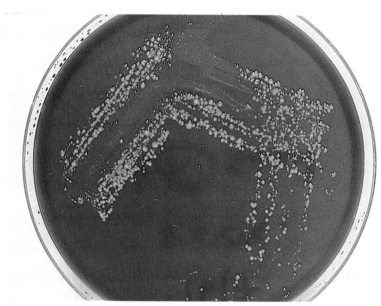

Plate 3 *Legionella pneumophila:* colony growth on BCYE agar, 72 hours.

Tyrrell, 1978; Weir *et al.*, 1982), changes in the central nervous system are minimal and the cerebrospinal fluid stays normal.

Animal models

An animal model for legionnaires' disease has been established particularly in guinea-pigs, rats and common marmosets (Baskerville *et al.*, 1981; Baskerville 1984; Winn *et al.*, 1982). Exposure to virulent *L. pneumophila* in small particle size aerosols (< 5 μm) results in fever and lobular broncho-pneumonia rapidly changing to lobar, with associated blood-stained pleural effusion and accompanied by considerable mortality. Histologically the pneumonia, showing alveoli distended with fibrinous exudate and cell debris containing macrophages and polymorphs resembles the human disease. Again, lesions in brain, liver, kidneys or other organs do not develop.

References

Baskerville, A. (1984). Pathology and Pathophysiology. In *Legionella: Proceedings of the 2nd International Symposium: Washington, DC.*, pp. 136–41. Edited by Thornsberry, C., Balows, A., Feeley, J.C. and Jakubowski, W. American Society for Microbiology, Washington.

Baskerville, A., Fitzgeorge, R.B., Broster, M. *et al.* (1981). Experimental transmission of Legionnaires' disease by exposure to aerosols of *Legionella pneumophila*. *Lancet* **2**, 1389–90.

Bernardini, D.L., Lerrick, K.S., Hoffman, K. and Lange, M. (1985). Neurogenic bladder: new clinical finding in Legionnaires' disease. *Am J Med* **78**, 1045–6.

Blackmon, J.A., Harley, R.A., Hicklin, M.D. and Chandler, F.W. (1979). Pulmonary sequelae of acute Legionnaires' disease pneumonia. *Ann Intern Med* **90**, 552–4.

Blackmon, J.A., Hicklin, M.D. and Chandler, F.W. (1978). Special Expert Pathology Panel. Legionnaires' disease; pathological and historical aspects of a 'new' disease. *Arch Pathol Lab Med* **102**, 337–43.

Boyd, J.F., Buchanan, W.M., MacLeod, T.I.F. *et al.* (1978). Pathology of five Scottish deaths from pneumonic illness acquired in Spain due to Legionnaires' disease agents. *J Clin Pathol* **31**, 809–16.

Brown, S.L., Bibb, W.F., and McKinney, R.M. (1985). Use of monoclonal antibodies in an epidemiological marker system: a retrospective study of lung specimens from the 1976 outbreak of Legionnaires' disease in Philadelphia by indirect fluorescent antibody and enzyme-linked immunosorbent assay methods. *J Clin Microbiol* **21**, 15–19.

Dournon, E., Bure, E., Kemeny, J.L. *et al.* (1982). *Legionella pneumophila* peritonitis. *Lancet* **1**, 1363.

Dowling, J.N., Kroboth, F.J., Karpf, M. *et al.* (1983). Pneumonia and multiple lung abscess caused by dual infection with *L. micdadei* and *L. pneumophila*. *Am Rev Resp Dis* **127**, 121–5.

Gatell, J.M., Miro, J.M., Sasal, M. *et al.* (1981). *Legionella pneumophila* antigen in brain. *Lancet* **2**, 202.

Hicklin, M.D., Thomason, B.M., Chandler, F.W. and Blackmon, J.A. (1980). Pathogenesis of acute Legionnaires' disease pneumonia. *Am J Clin Path* **73**, 480–87.

Lees, A.W. and Tyrrell, W.F. (1978). Severe cerebral disturbance in Legionnaires' disease. *Lancet* **2**, 1336-7.

McCabe, R.E., Baldwin, J.C., McGregor, C.A. *et al.* (1984). Prosthetic valve endocarditis caused by *Legionella pneumophila*. *Ann Intern Med* **100**, 525-7.

Macfarlane, J.T., Miller, A.C., Morris, A.H. *et al.* (1984). Comparative radiographic features of Legionnaires' disease and other sporadic community acquired pneumonias. In *Legionella: Proceedings of the 2nd International Symposium: Washington, DC.*, pp. 12-13. American Society for Microbiology, Washington.

Maycock, R., Skale, B. and Kohler, R.B. (1983). Legionella pneumophila pericarditis proved by culture of pericardial fluid. *Am J Med* **75**, 534-6.

Nelson, D.P., Rensimer, E.R. and Raffin, T.A. (1985). *Legionella pneumophila* pericarditis without pneumonia. *Arch Intern Med* **145**, 926.

Rodgers, F.G. (1979). Ultrastructure of *Legionella pneumophila*. *J Clin Pathol* **32**, 1195-202.

Rodgers, F.G. (1983). The role of structure and invasiveness on the pathogenicity of Legionella. *Zbl Bakt Hyg I Abt Orig A* **255**, 138-44.

Schlanger, G., Lutwick, L.I., Kurzman, M. *et al.* (1984). Sinusitis caused by Legionella pneumophila in a patient with the acquired immune deficiency syndrome. *Am J Med* **77**, 957-60.

Weir, A.I., Bone, I. and Kennedy, D.H. (1982). Neurological involvement in legionellosis. *J Neurol Neurosurg Pyschiat* **45**, 603-8.

Weisenberger, D.D., Helms, C.M. and Renner, E.D. (1981). Sporadic Legionnaires' disease. A pathologic study of 23 fatal cases. *Arch Pathol Lab Med* **105**, 130-7.

White, H.J., Felton, W. and Sun, C.N. (1980). Extrapulmonary histopathologic manifestations of Legionnaires' disease. Evidence for myocarditis and bacteremia. *Arch Pathol Lab Med* **104**, 287-9.

Winn, W.C., Davis, G.S. Gump, D.W. *et al.* (1982). Legionnaires' pneumonia after intratracheal inoculation of guinea pigs and rats. *Lab Invest* **47**, 568-78.

Winn, W.C. and Myerowitz, R.L. (1981). The pathology of Legionella pneumonias. *Human Pathol* **12**, 401-22.

6 Laboratory Diagnosis

The accurate and early identification of aetiological organisms, is important in severe microbial infections both for effective treatment and on epidemiological grounds. In this, legionellosis is no exception. Since the causative microorganism was first described (McDade *et al.*, 1977) and named *Legionella pneumophila* (Brenner *et al.*, 1979), it has become a prototype for numerous phenotypic bacteria whose unique features have led to their grouping within the new family of Legionellaceae. This now includes at least 23 legionella species with eleven serogroups of *L. pneumophila* and two serogroups for each of the species, *L. bozemanii*, *L. longbeachae*, *L. feeleii* and *L. hackeliae* (Bercovier *et al.*, 1986; Brenner, 1984; Brenner *et al.*, 1985; Edelstein *et al.*, 1984). Many of these have been associated with human disease.

In both sporadic incidents and outbreaks of legionella infection the predominant clinical feature has mostly been a form of pneumonia, often innocuous initially but on occasion developing into a severe and, at times, fatal illness. Although severe pneumonia commonly results from pneumococcal infection, *Mycoplasma pneumoniae*, legionella species and other organisms are also in contention (Macfarlane *et al.*, 1982). Laboratory assistance in determining aetiology and in monitoring progress is therefore important. Preliminary laboratory investigations such as the haematological, biochemical and other reactions of legionnaires' disease are dealt with in Chapter 3.

Non-pneumonic manifestations of legionella infection which have been reported include Pontiac fever (Fraser *et al.*, 1979; Glick *et al.*, 1978; Herwaldt *et al.*, 1984), renal failure (Kerr *et al.*, 1978; Wegmüller *et al.*, 1985), haemolytic anaemia (Strikas *et al.*, 1983), neurological complications including cerebral, cerebellar or brain stem involvement (Bernardini *et al.*, 1985; Johnson *et al.*, 1984; Lees and Tyrrell, 1978; Pearson and Dadds, 1981), peritonitis (Dournon *et al.*, 1982), perirectal abscess (Arnow *et al.*, 1983), cutaneous abscess (Ampel *et al.*, 1985), haemodialysis fistula infection (Kalweit *et al.*, 1982), wound infection (Brabender *et al.*, 1983), sinusitis (Schlanger *et al.*, 1984) and pericarditis (Nelson *et al.*, 1985).

Implication of a particular organism as a cause of disease requires at least one but preferably all of the following steps.

(a) Recognition of the organism in body fluids, exudates, biopsy material or post-mortem tissues in which it would not ordinarily be present.

(b) Growth of the organism from such specimens by inoculation of extracts into experimental animals, embryonated hens' eggs, or on to appropriate culture media.

(c) Search for specific antigens or toxins released by the organisms, any of which may be present in body fluids, exudates or tissue extracts.

(d) Identification retrospectively in sera of specific humoral responses to the organisms by the body's defensive immune system.

Clinical material

With pneumonia as the predominant manifestation, specimens from the lower respiratory tract are required as follows.

Sputum	Expectorated sample or from tracheal suction. Specimens may be difficult to obtain during the early stage of illness but physiotherapy sometimes helps. The recovery of legionella species from sputum of patients with pneumonia by use of selective media has become more frequent and should now be routinely attempted. Inability to culture such organisms from the oropharynx of asymptomatic adults adds to the significance of successful isolation (Edelstein, 1983).
Tracheal aspirate	Obtained by transtracheal aspiration or injection of saline (Macfarlane and Ward, 1984). Such aspirates have been claimed to be the optimal source for the recovery of legionella (Zuravleff *et al.*, 1983).
Bronchial aspirate	Obtained by bronchoscopy including bronchoalveolar lavage. This is not yet used routinely but can lead to more rapid diagnosis as well as increasing the isolation rate of organisms (Winter *et al.*, 1986).
Pleural exudate	Obtained by needle tap. Pleural fluid provided an early isolate of *L. pneumophila* (Dumoff, 1979) but culture yields may be low compared to other sources (Edelstein, 1983). Whether specific antigens may be present needs further study.
Lung biopsies	Percutaneous needle aspirate; transbronchoscopic or open lung biopsy. May be of value if done early, especially in immunocompromised patients but is not usually required (Matthay and Moritz, 1981).
Autopsy specimens	Consolidated lung tissue. Extrathoracic sites particularly spleen, kidneys, bone marrow (Weisenburger *et al.*, 1980; JAMA, 1980).
Blood culture	The varying manifestations of legionellosis suggest that blood spread of organisms occurs, though the low recovery rate contrasts with the situation in pneumococcal infection. To account for this the organisms

(a) May not be in the circulation when blood samples are withdrawn.

(b) May be intracellular in monocytes and macrophages

being dealt with by the body's protective mechanisms which impede release.

(c) May be inhibited by the culture media used.

Urine   Centrifuged deposit for culture or detection of specific antigen in supernate by a number of serological methods. Concentration of supernate may be required.

CSF   If abnormal, test for specific antigens as per urine.

Serum   For retrospective development of specific antibodies. These may appear 1–2 weeks after the onset of illness or may be delayed till later. It is therefore essential to any investigation that sequential samples are collected from hospital admission to late convalescence.

Table 6.1 shows tests commonly applied to specimens from patients.

Environmental specimens   See Chapter 8. Water samples in general need to be concentrated, usually by filtration, before further investigation; this makes prior arrangement advisable.

Microscopy

For the detection of organisms in the secretions or tissues of a patient, microscopic examination is desirable, the methods ranging from non-specific to specific. Materials should include liquefied sputum (not saliva), tracheal or bronchial aspirates, pleural fluids and lung tissue extracts either fresh or formolized. Such materials should be handled with aseptic precautions due to their possible pathogen content and because of the need also for culture and storage. Smears, prepared by spreading small amounts of material on clean glass slides are air-dried, gently heat-fixed and acetone treated. With consolidated lung a freshly cut surface, scraped with a scalpel blade and the material emulsified in distilled water or saline, gives good preparations in diagnosing legionella infections.

The purpose of staining is two-fold, both to observe the cellular response to the inflammation and to look for organisms. Large numbers of polymorphonuclear leucocytes, particularly in sputum, are associated with pneumococcal infections whereas in legionellosis cells are fewer in number, comprising a mixture of polymorphs and monocytes, the latter often predominating. A Gram stain will differentiate Gram-positive organisms such as *Streptococcus pneumoniae* from those which are Gram-negative such as *Haemophilus influenzae* or the legionella group. Because legionellas may stain poorly, prolongation of staining time and the use of basic fuchsin as the counterstain has been recommended. The initial application of the half-a-Gram stain (De Freitas *et al.*, 1979) may sometimes be helpful.

The morphological appearance of *L. pneumophila* found in patients' secretions or tissues is of a small Gram-negative coccobacillary rod with non-parallel sides and tapered ends. When cultured, particularly on suboptimal media, non-dividing elongated to filamentous forms, often with vacuoles, may be found. In addition to Gram, other stains used have been Giemsa, Gimenez and Sudan black B for fat droplets.

Table 6.1 Legionella investigations

Material	Preparation	Stain	Electron microscopy	Culture	Organism identification
1. Sputum	(i) Smears of emulsified sputum, heat-fixed on slide (ii) Smears as above but additionally acetone treated	Gram counterstained with dilute carbol-fuchsin 3–5 minutes. Fluorescent antibody (b1) direct conjugate for each serogroup *or* (b2) monoclonal antibody conjugate against all *L. pneumophila* serogroups. *or* (b3) indirect sandwich test with antisera to each serogroup or species	If Gram-negative rods present, examine by negative staining. Useful only when large numbers of organisms present	Sputum inoculation on buffered CYE agar with α-ketoglutarate plus antibiotics. Use moist plates, CO_2 incubator preferable. Examine plates after 48 hours then daily for 7–8 days. Discard as negative after 14–21 days. Examine all suspect colonies by staining and subculture. Species other than *L. pneumophila* may take more than 7 days to grow	Fluorescent antibody test with available serogroup antisera. For further confirmation, send to specialist laboratory
2. Aspirate (i) tracheal } (ii) bronchial }	Smears as for Sputum	Gram if sufficient material available. Try centrifugation to obtain deposit for examination. FAT even if Gram-negative rods not seen.	*See above*	BCYE agar *as above*	*See above* if suspected colonies seen
3. Lung (ante-mortem) (i) percutaneous puncture (ii) open biopsy	*See above*	Gram, if sufficient material, FAT similarly	Thin section EM after glutaraldehyde fixation of small portion of tissue	BCYE agar, as above, from unfixed material	*See above*

4. Lung- (post-mortem)	(i) impression smears on slide of freshly cut lung surface heat-fixed,	Gram	Thin section EM after glutaraldehyde fixation of small portion of tissue	BCYE agar as above from unfixed material	*See above*
	(ii) acetone treated for FAT			
	(iii) emulsified suspension of scraping from cut consolidated area, heat or formol-fixed	Gram		
	(iv) acetone treated for FAT			
5. Other exudates or tissues	When practicable apply any or all above techniques			*See above*
6. Blood culture	As in other acute illnesses; when legionella suspected an enriched yeast extract broth containing L-cysteine and soluble ferric pyrophosphate may be inoculated also Subculture both after 7 days on to BCYE agar and examine plates as above			
7. Sera	Collect early (1–7 days) intermediate (10–20 days) and convalescent (6 weeks) samples. These may be stored frozen while awaiting tests. It is useful to divide into aliquots to avoid repeated freezing and thawing			
8. Antigens	Sputum or urine may contain group-specific antigens. Store specimens frozen pending investigation by IEOP, ELISA, RIA etc			

The specific identification of legionella serogroups and species is still done mainly by the fluorescent antibody staining technique utilizing high-titre and more recently monoclonal antisera. When such antisera have been directly fluorescein-conjugated the test is completed in a single stage. This was an advantage when few *L. pneumophila* serogroups were known and most clinical infections attributable to serogroup 1. It has again become effective with a monoclonal antibody directed against a common bacterial outer membrane protein (Tenover *et al.*, 1985). The ever increasing number of new serogroups however, plus the production of highly-specific monoclonal antibodies makes the two stage technique more applicable. In this, the conjugated antisera are applied first to smears, the excess removed by washing and then an overlay of the appropriate fluorescent conjugated anti-animal-species globulin is applied.

Identification of Gram-negative organisms found in secretions, tissues or after culture may be aided by electron microscopic examination of negatively stained material. With legionella species the characteristic outline of these organisms has been shown, also their occurrence both intra and extra-cellularly, their possession of flagella and fimbriae and their specific identification by an immunoferritin technique (Rodgers, 1979, 1983).

Bacterial culture

With pneumonia, identification of the likely pathogen as quickly as possible is an aid to effective treatment. Laboratory investigations should, therefore, include aerobic and anaerobic cultivation of available material on solid and in fluid media. Among well-known potential causative organisms are *S. pneumoniae*, *H. influenzae*, *M. pneumoniae* and now the legionella group with which we are mainly concerned. The legionellas are small, slow growing, Gram-negative organisms. They need L-cysteine and possibly iron salts in growth media and are apt to be inhibited or suppressed by saline solutions, substances in the saliva or tissues and can be smothered by other more rapidly growing bacteria. The use of selective media and careful application of heat and/or acid treatment to impede bacterial contaminants should increase the possibility of recovery from specimens.

Because of difficulties due to the unknown nature of the organisms, *L. pneumophila*, the first isolate of the species, was recovered by guinea-pig intraperitoneal inoculation followed by subculture of peritoneal exudate in the yolk sacs of fertile hens' eggs (McDade *et al.*, 1977). Not only was the guinea-pig susceptible by this route but other contaminating organisms were often suppressed during the time of legionella multiplication, providing virtually pure cultures for inoculation into the yolk sacs. Though effective, this technique had some limitations to its use (Bopp *et al.*, 1981) and appears less sensitive than direct culture on selective media (Fitzgeorge and Dennis, 1983). Weaver (1978) reported the successful transfer of the organisms to supplemented Mueller-Hinton agar medium though growth occurred comparatively slowly. Analysis of the medium supplements showed L-cysteine hydrochloride to be essential for growth and iron salts such as ferric pyrophosphate highly desirable. These ingredients are now routinely incorporated into legionella culture media.

New media which were better able to support growth of legionellas were quickly introduced (Feeley *et al.*, 1978). Small colonies presenting a cut-glass appearance were found to grow on a clear medium (Feeley-Gorman or F-G agar) containing casein hydrolysate, starch and beef extract. A brown melanin-related pigment also developed from oxidation of tyrosine in areas surrounding heavy growth. Yeast-extract tyrosine agar has also been found useful for this (Bopp *et al.*, 1981). When viewed in long wave ultraviolet light the colonies showed a yellowish fluorescence. Such characteristics of the *L. pneumophila* group can help to distinguish them from other species. Introduced about the same time, a CYE agar medium (Feeley *et al.*, 1979) was felt to be more sensitive than F-G agar for legionella culture including primary isolation though, being opaque, it could not show pigment formation, (see Plate 3). Other growth requirements included a narrow pH range centred on 6.9, the presence of CO_2 (2–5 per cent), an optimal incubation temperature of 35°C within the range 25–42°C, and a high relative humidity. To begin with, adjustment of the pH to 6.9 was with NaOH but it was soon noted that an excess of sodium in the presence of charcoal could be inhibitory to the organisms. Alteration of the medium by adding N-2-acetamido-2-amino-ethane sulfonic acid (ACES) buffer and adjusting to pH 6.9 with KOH instead, resulted in greater sensitivity (Pasculle *et al.*, 1980) as did the addition of α-ketoglutarate though not selenium (Edelstein, 1981). With these improvements the need to incubate cultures in the presence of CO_2 was less necessary.

Culture of legionella species from both patient material and environmental sources is now practicable in many microbiological laboratories, particularly since media became available commercially. Problems of recognition do exist due to their slow delicate growth, the presence in certain clinical and environmental samples of contaminating faster growing organisms and the lack of suitable chemical enzymic reactions to distinguish new isolates. To increase medium selectivity inclusion of antimicrobial agents such as amphotericin B, anisomycin, cefamandole, colistin, polymyxin B, trimethoprim and vancomysin has been advocated. Glycine, being an inhibitor of many Gram-negative organisms (Wadowsky and Yee, 1981) and cyclohexamide for its antifungal effect (Bopp *et al.*, 1981; Fitzgeorge and Dennis 1983) are other favoured inclusions.

For the investigation of clinical material, Edelstein (1983) favoured a buffered CYE agar supplemented with α-ketoglutarate, anisomycin for its antifungal effect, cefamandole and polymyxin B. This is effective against yeasts, commensal and enteric bacteria though not against pseudomonas and serratia species or group D streptococci. Should pseudomonads be a problem a cephalosporin such as ceftazidime could however be tried. This medium may be inhibitory to some legionellas including *L. micdadei*. An alternative medium, useful in environmental studies but inactive against common Gram-negative organisms, was a buffered CYE agar containing α-ketoglutarate, glycine, vancomycin and polymyxin B as supplements. Though effective, antimicrobials in culture media may delay the appearance of the legionella colonies.

By adding dyes such as bromocresol purple and bromothymol blue (Vickers *et al.*, 1981) or aniline blue (Holmes, 1982) to culture media, colour and fluorescence changes were added to colonial appearance as presumptive markers between species though this did not eliminate the need for specific identification. Newly isolated strains should be fully investigated to ensure that such features are not variable.

Among alternative culture media, horse blood agar, enriched with L-cysteine and iron salts and made selective by adding amphotericin B, colistin, trimethoprim and vancomycin, supported the growth of legionella species both for primary isolation and passage (Greaves, 1980). Reducing the sodium chloride content further enhanced its sensitivity (Dennis *et al.*, 1981). When compared with buffered CYE agar the Greaves (1980) medium was found to be less sensitive (Keathley and Winn, 1984), but its modification in 1981 appeared to make it considerably more effective (Kaan and MacLaren, 1986).

That legionella species are present may be confirmed by culture on media with or without L-cysteine. On the latter, growth should not ordinarily occur. Only *L. oakridgensis* and *L. jordanis* have been found capable of doing so after passage (Edelstein, 1983). As an alternative, (Smith, 1982) applied L-cysteine impregnated discs to the medium lacking it and looked for characteristic growth in the vicinity of the discs.

Bacteraemia, particularly in the severely ill, is common during the early pyrexial phase of pneumonia, blood culture being a standard procedure. Recovery of legionella organisms, however, has been infrequent despite clinical evidence of manifestations outside the respiratory system. Transparent liquid media containing L-cysteine and iron salts and capable of supporting growth of such organisms have been devised (Edelstein, 1983; Greaves, 1980; Johnson *et al.*, 1982). Whether such substances should always be incorporated in blood culture media would depend on the likely frequency of sporadic legionellosis and on their not suppressing the growth of other pathogens. Chester and his colleagues (1983) noted a successful isolation of *L. pneumophila* even after 7 days incubation in an aerobic blood culture bottle, then subcultured on to legionella supportive solid medium. Survival of the organisms at least, if not actual multiplication, must have occurred. Further studies of this procedure also proved successful (Rihs *et al.*, 1985).

Pre-treatment of environmental specimens

Steps to prevent or reduce the growth of other organisms have included the use of a low pH or heat to pre-treat specimens. *L. pneumophila* survived briefly in conditions down to pH2 (Wang *et al.*, 1979) and, based on this, methods for preliminary acid treatment of suspensions have been described (Edelstein, 1983; Greaves, 1980; Bopp *et al.*, 1981). Though the technique of mixing aliquots of suspension and acid (HC1 pH2) or acid buffer (HC1/KC1 pH 2.2) for a short period then neutralizing the mixture can be useful in reducing contaminants, such treatment also tends to reduce the viable count of legionella organisms and may be ineffective when only small numbers are present initially.

Legionella organisms are widely present in the water systems of large buildings (Bartlett *et al.*, 1986; Lancet, 1983). They can multiply even in tap water between 25°C and 42°C (Yee and Wadowsky, 1982) and appear able to survive for varying periods at temperatures ranging from 15°C–55°C or even higher, being more resistant in this respect than most other environmental organisms. Because of this, pre-treatment of suspensions at 50°C for 30 minutes (Dennis *et al.*, 1984) or 60°C for 3 minutes (Edelstein, 1983) has been advocated.

Characterization of organisms

Identification of suspected legionella organisms should include their biochemical reactions, an ever increasing range of serological tests, DNA relatedness tests among species, analysis by gas liquid chromatography (GLC) of their branched chain fatty acids, and by thin-layer chromatography of their quinones (Karr *et al.*, 1982; Tang *et al.*, 1984). The biochemical reactions, summarized by Fallon (1981) show a lack of carbohydrate fermentation with variation in gelatin liquefaction, oxidase, catalase, pigment formation, β-lactamase production and sodium hippurate hydrolysis (Hébert, 1981). The enzymatic profile as in the AP1-ZYM system may be utilized (Müller, 1981; Nolte *et al.*, 1982).

Serological identification is most specific, allowing separation into species and groups. A macroscopic slide agglutination test introduced by Wilkinson and Fikes (1980) has been developed into a means of identifying all known species and serogroups (Thacker *et al.*, 1985). It makes use of antisera rendered specific by absorption of any cross-reacting elements. Such antisera may then be used individually or in the form of overlapping pools. The established method has been the fluorescent antibody test (Cherry *et al.*, 1978). Though done initially with directly conjugated antiserum it has now become more usual to apply the indirect sandwich technique. Although this method is usually without major problems, cross-reactions with non-legionella organisms such as some strains of pseudomonas and bacteroides species have been reported (Orrison *et al.*, 1983).

Confirmation of the identity of legionella species is obtainable from analysis by chromatography of their cellular lipids. These, present mainly in the bacterial outer membrane, are made up of branched chain fatty acids and long chain isoprenoid quinones (Collins and Gilbart, 1983; Moss *et al.*, 1983). Species have their distinctive profiles. The techniques of gas liquid chromatography are likely to be done only in certain reference laboratories.

Direct identification of legionella in specimens by hydridization with a radiolabelled deoxyribonucleic acid (DNA) probe has been proposed but no details given (Kohne *et al.*, 1984; Shaw *et al.*, 1985). A DNA probe deprived of cross-hybridizing fragments and thus specific for *L. pneumophila* has also been described (Grimont *et al.*, 1985). While such probes may confirm the presence of legionellas in patient or environmental material, precise identification of the organisms will probably need additional serological or cultural techniques.

As with other pneumonias when circumstances such as prior antibiotic therapy or late admission to hospital render detection of the causative organism by staining or culture difficult, it may still be possible to detect soluble specific antigen from the organism in sputum or urine. Tests for this include counter-immune electrophoresis (CIE) radio-immune assay (RIA), enzyme-linked immunosorbent assay (ELISA) or latex agglutination. Understandably, the more complicated tests such as RIA or ELISA may be more sensitive, providing a higher ratio of positive results but a single agglutination test utilizing antibody-coated latex particles can be almost as effective (Sathapatayavongs *et al.*, 1983). Furthermore, such rapid diagnostic techniques are still not widely used.

The role of serology

Since the aetiology of the disease was established in late 1977, diagnosis has mostly been serological in legionella pneumonia. Despite the advent of more satisfactory media for isolating the organisms (Edelstein, 1984) serology is still a mainstay. Its disadvantage is that antibody determination has to be retrospective. The body's immune mechanisms become demonstrable only when the affected person has survived the first few days of illness. The development of antibody can then be followed during the period to convalescence and its persistence beyond that also measured. The simplest demonstration, therefore, of an association between organism and disease is a rising antibody titre, four-fold or greater, to the organisms during the course of the illness. This needs a minimum of two spaced serum samples, though further sequential specimens can be helpful. The first of these should be taken as soon as possible after the onset. If obtained within 3–5 days it should be virtually devoid of antibody and, although not of immediate help to the clinician, it can establish a base line against which later results may be compared. However, in the rush of admitting a seriously ill patient to hospital an early blood sample for serology may not always be taken. Should admission have been delayed a number of days because of home treatment the lack of a specific bacterial isolate also means that sera have to be tested against a range of serogroups and species.

Because legionella antibodies may develop relatively early, for example within 6–8 days from the apparent onset of illness, or else be delayed until the 3rd week, suitably spaced serum samples are vital to the diagnosis. Should the clinical manifestations be at all suggestive a diagnosis should not be ruled out unless a late convalescent stage serum sample (6 weeks) has been found negative. A high antibody titre (e.g. $\geqslant 256$) in a single late sample may, on occasion, be acceptable as diagnostic though it is suggestive more than absolute. Some patients retain high circulating antibody titres for months or even years though it is uncertain whether this reflects a persisting focus of infection. It may be helpful to study the circulating immune globulin classes M, G and A, in particular specific immunoglobulin M (IgM) and immunoglobulin G (IgG). As in other diseases the IgM usually appears early, accounting for most of the measurable antibody to begin with. During convalescence it declines, being replaced by IgG which can then persist for years either as a stable entity or show a gradual recession. Variations have, however, been reported; on occasion only IgM has been found, at other times virtually only IgG. When present it is accepted that, for the most part, IgM signifies current or recent infection whereas IgG alone may be an indicator of past infection. IgA may also be found in recent infection but is liable to rapid degradation (Wilkinson *et al.*, 1983).

Another variable feature is the mode of antibody development. Among many patients the response has been found strictly serogroup specific. Others show a broader type of response with a rise in titre to more than one *L. pneumophila* serogroup or even to separate legionella species. This could result from a dual infection as instances of this have been reported (Joly and Winn, 1984). It may, however, simply reflect stimulation of surface or core antigens common to the species, of common flagellar antigen (Brenner *et al.*, 1985; Rodgers and Laverick, 1984), or even of antigens in common with other Gram-negative organisms. Sometimes the dilemma can be clarified when the homologous antibody response is greater than others. Alternatively cross-absorption tests may be done though these are time-consuming and specialist techniques (Wilkinson *et al.*, 1983).

Despite the many new species of Legionellaceae being identified (Brenner, 1984; Brenner *et al.*, 1985) the organism largely responsible for severe human disease is still *L. pneumophila* serogroup 1. The factors providing it with such virulence are, however, still under investigation. Within species the existence of separate serogroups and, particularly for *L. pneumophila* serogroup 1 of at least eleven major subgroups has been reported (Joly and Winn, 1984; Joly *et al.*, 1986; Para and Plouffe, 1983; Watkins and Tobin, 1984; Watkins *et al.*, 1985) so that a correct serological diagnosis with standard antigens may not necessarily be made. Should an isolate from the patient be available when the routine test is equivocal, a more clear-cut result may be obtained by the use of the patient's own organism as antigen or by subgrouping it. Serological overlap between legionella species and organisms such as *Mycoplasma pneumoniae* or *Chlamydia psittaci* had at one stage been postulated but is now thought unlikely (Edelstein, 1984; Taylor *et al.*, 1980).

Serological confirmation of the diagnosis of legionellosis is now possible by other procedures but none has, as yet, replaced on any scale the indirect fluorescent antibody test. Fears that results from this test might not be comparable between laboratories have been largely overcome by the adoption of standardized methods and reagents and by quality control of results, including specificity (Taylor and Harrison, 1983). Some controversy has existed over methods for preparing antigens either by heat-fixation (Fallon and Abraham, 1982; Wilkinson *et al.*, 1981) or by dilute formalin fixation (Taylor and Harrison, 1981). It would appear both methods provide effective diagnostic antigens (Wilkinson and Brake, 1982) though Taylor and Harrison (1981, 1983) believe there are fewer non-specific reactions with formolized antigens. With the increasing number of serogroups and species antigen pools are now used for preliminary screening.

For these tests, acceptable diagnostic criteria, now established and time-honoured, consist of a four-fold or greater antibody rise in titre e.g. from below 16 to 64 or more, the figures being reciprocals of the original serum dilutions under examination. A single convalescent phase serum must have a titre of 128 or more, in conjunction with pneumonia, to be considered a probable diagnosis, particularly when this is strengthened by the presence of specific IgM. Finding IgG alone, even in high titre particularly if it remains unchanged will mostly signify a past infection.

Minor difficulties over fluorescence and the fact that legionellas can be specifically agglutinated have led to the micro-agglutination test for antibody estimation (Farshy *et al.*, 1978) and its projection as a rapid and simple alternative method (Harrison and Taylor, 1982, 1984). Its sensitivity in terms of current infection with *L. pneumophila* serogroup 1 has been claimed to parallel the fluorescent antibody test with the proviso that it measures the IgM antibody and is not likely to detect any IgG antibody present. Apart from its relatively restricted scale of use, and this applies also in other serological tests, one problem is the preparation and distribution to diagnostic laboratories of tried and tested antigens.

An enzyme-linked immunosorbent assay (ELISA) which utilizes soluble or EDTA-extract antigen from legionella species adsorbed to polystyrene microtitre plates or cuvettes can provide an alternative test to fluorescence (Farshy *et al.*, 1978; Wreghitt *et al.*, 1982; Zuravleff *et al.*, 1983). In essence, the test is similar, in that antibody from a patient's serum is bound to the antigen coating. The bound antibody is then conjoined to enzyme-linked antihuman globulin which may be IgM, IgG or a combination. Its amount can be measured after the addition of an appropriate substrate. This is done either visually from colour change or more exactly by spectrophotometric print-out. It is claimed to be a sensitive and specific test. The technique may however be less suitable than fluorescence or micro-agglutination for small numbers of tests.

A further test for antibody measurement is the indirect haemagglutination test with the antigens adsorbed to turkey erythrocytes (Yonke *et al.*, 1981). Antigen detection in urine has been reported by a reverse passive haemagglutination test (Tang *et al.*, 1982), by RIA (Kohler *et al.*, 1981) by latex agglutination (Sathapatayavongs *et al.*, 1983) and by ELISA (Bibb *et al.*, 1984).

Safety in laboratories

Although legionella species are widely distributed in nature, no convincing evidence for person-to-person spread has been elicited. Nonetheless they can on occasion act as pathogens particularly as a result of inhalation. Therefore, in the diagnostic laboratory all suspect material for investigation should be handled with care in accordance at least with World Health Organization (WHO) risk category 2 for hospital pathogens. In Britain, the Advisory Committee on Dangerous Pathogens in 1984 recommended that the legionellaceae be categorized in hazard group 2. When stored in a moist state organisms can remain viable for several days at a temperature of 4°C. Material for long term preservation should, however, be kept at a temperature of − 70°C or lower. Sera are least likely to deteriorate when frozen at or below − 70°C though when there are problems of space, temperatures of − 40°C to − 30°C may be acceptable.

References

Advisory Committee on Dangerous Pathogens (1984). *Categorization of Pathogens According to Hazard and Categories of Containment.* HMSO. London.

Ampel, N.M., Ruben, F.L. and Norden, C.W. (1985). Cutaneous abscess caused by *Legionella micdadei* in an immunosuppressed patient. *Ann Intern Med* **102**, 630–32.

Arnow, P.M., Boyko, E.J. and Friedman, E.L. (1983). Perirectal abscess caused by *Legionella pneumophila* and mixed anaerobic bacteria. *Ann Intern Med* **98**, 184–5.

Bartlett, C.L.R., Dennis, P.J.L., Harper, D. *et al.* (1986). Legionella in plumbing systems. Submitted for publication.

Bercovier, H., Steigerwalt, A.G., Derhi-Cochin, M. *et al.* (1986). Isolation of legionellae from oxidation ponds and fishponds in Israel and description of *Legionella israelensis* sp. nov. *Int J Syst Bact* **36**, 368–71.

Bernardini, D.L., Lerrick, K.S., Hoffman, K. and Lange, M. (1985). Neurogenic bladder: new clinical finding in Legionnaires' disease. *Am J Med* **78**, 1045–6.

Bibb, W.F., Arnow, P.M., Thacker, L. and McKinney, R.M. (1984). Detection of soluble *Legionella pneumophila* antigens in serum and urine specimens by enzyme-linked immunosorbent assay with monoclonal and polyclonal antibodies. *J Clin Microbiol* **20**, 478–82.

Bopp, C.A., Sumner, J.W., Morris, G.K. and Wells, J.G. (1981). Isolation of *Legionella* spp. from environmental water samples by low pH treatment and use of a selective medium. *J Clin Microbiol* **13**, 714–19.

Brabender, W., Hinthorn, D.R., Asher, M. *et al.*, (1983). *Legionella pneumophila* wound infection. *JAMA* **250**, 3091–2.

Brenner, D.J. (1984). Classification of Legionellae. In *Legionella: Proceedings of the 2nd International Symposium: Washington, DC.*, pp. 55–60. Edited by Thornsberry, C., Balows, A., Feeley, J.C. and Jakubowski, W. American Society for Microbiology, Washington.

Brenner, D.J., Steigerwalt, A.G., Gorman, G.W. *et al.* (1985). Ten new species of *Legionella*. *Int J Syst Bact* **35**, 50–59.

Brenner, D.J., Steigerwalt, A.G., McDade, J.E. (1979). Classification of the Legion-naires' disease bacterium: *Legionella pneumophila*, genus novum, species, nova, of the family Legionellaceae, familia nova. *Ann Intern Med* **90**, 656–8.

Cherry, W.B., Pittman, B., Harris P.P. *et al.*, (1978). Detection of Legionnaires' disease bacteria by direct immunofluorescent staining. *J Clin Microbiol* **8**, 329–38.

Chester, B., Poulos, E.G., Demaray, M.J. *et al.* (1983). Isolation of *Legionella pneumophila* serogroup 1 from blood with nonsupplemented blood culture bottles. *J Clin Microbiol* **17**, 195–7.

Collins, M.D. Gilbart, J. (1983). New members of the coenzyme Q series from the Legionellaceae. *FEMS Microbiol Lett* **16**, 251–5.

De Freitas, J.L., Borst, J, and Meenhorst, P.L. (1979). Easy visualization of *Legionella pneumophila* by 'half-a-gram' stain procedure. *Lancet* **1**, 27–71.

Dennis, P.J., Bartlett, C.L.R. and Wright, A.E. (1984). Comparison of isolation methods for *Legionella* spp. In *Legionella: Proceedings of the 2nd International Symposium: Washington, DC.*, pp. 294–6. Edited by Thornsberry, C., Balows, A., Feeley, J.C. and Jakubowski, W. American Society for Microbiology, Washington.

Dennis, P.J., Taylor, J.A. and Barrow, G.I. (1981). Phosphate buffered, low sodium chloride blood agar medium for *Legionella pneumophila*. *Lancet* **2**, 636.

Dournon, E., Bure, A., Kemeny, J.L. *et al.* (1982). *Legionella pneumophila* peritonitis. *Lancet* **1**, 1363.

Dumoff, M. (1979). Direct *in-vitro* isolation of the Legionnaires' disease bacterium in two fatal cases. *Ann Intern Med* **90**, 694–6.

Edelstein, P.H. (1981). Improved semi-selective medium for isolation of *Legionella pneumophila* from contaminated clinical and environmental specimens. *J Clin Microbiol* **14**, 298–303.

Edelstein, P.H. (1983). Culture diagnosis of Legionella infections. *Zbl Bakt Hyg I Abt Orig A* **255**, 96–101.

Edelstein, P.H. (1984). Laboratory diagnosis of Legionnaires' disease. In *Legionella: Proceedings of the 2nd International Symposium: Washington, DC.*, pp. 3–5. Edited by Thornsberry, C., Balows, A., Feeley, J.C. and Jakubowski, W. American Society for Microbiology, Washington.

Edelstein, P.H., Bibb, W.F., Gorman, G.W. *et al.* (1984). *Legionella pneumophila* serogroup 9: a cause of human pneumonia. *Ann Intern Med* **101** 196–8.

Fallon, R.J. (1981). Laboratory diagnosis of Legionnaires' disease. *ACP Broadsheet* **No. 99**.

Fallon, R.J. and Abraham, W.H. (1982). Polyvalent heat-killed antigen for the diagnosis of infection with *Legionella pneumophila*. *J Clin Pathol* **35**, 434–8.

Farshy, C.E., Klein, G.C. and Feeley, J.C. (1978). Detection of antibodies to Legionnaires' disease organism by microagglutination and microenzyme linked immunosorbent assay tests. *J Clin Microbiol* **7**, 327–31.

Feeley, J.C., Gibson, R.J., Gorman, G.W. *et al.* (1979). Charcoal-yeast extract agar: primary isolation medium for *Legionella pneumophila*. *J Clin Microbiol* **10**, 437–41.

Feeley, J.C., Gorman, G.W., Weaver, R.E. *et al.* (1978). Primary isolation media for the Legionnaires' disease bacterium. *J Clin Microbiol* **8**, 320–35.

Fitzgeorge, R.B. and Dennis, P.J. (1983). Isolation of *Legionella pneumophila* from water supplies: comparison of methods based on the guinea-pig and culture media. *J Hyg*, Camb **91**: 179–87.

Fraser, D.W., Deubner, D.C., Hill, D.L. and Gilliam, D.K. (1979). Nonpneumonic short incubation period legionellas (Pontiac fever) in men who cleaned a steam turbine condenser. *Science* **205**, 690–91.

Glick, T.H., Gregg, M.B., Berman, B. *et al.* (1978). An epidemic of unknown etiology in a health department: 1. Clinical and epidemiologic aspects. *Am J Epidemiol* **107**, 149–60.

Greaves, P.W. (1980). New methods for the isolation of *Legionella pneumophila*. *J Clin Pathol* **33**, 581–4.

Grimont, P.A.D., Grimont, F., Desplaces, N. and Tchen, P. (1985). DNA probe specific for *Legionella pneumophila*. *J Clin Microbiol* **21**, 431–7.

Harrison, T.G., and Taylor, A.G. (1982). A rapid microagglutination test for the diagnosis of *Legionella pneumophila* (serogroup 1) infection. *J Clin Pathol* **35**, 1028–31.

Harrison, T.G. and Taylor, A.G. (1984). Rapid microagglutination test and early diagnosis of Legionnaires' disease. In *Legionella: Proceedings of the 2nd International Symposium: Washington, DC.*, pp. 37–8. American Society for Microbiology, Washington.

Hébert, G.A. (1981). Hippurate hydrolysis by *Legionella pneumophila*. *J Clin Microbiol* **13**, 240–42.

Herwaldt, L.A., Gorman, G.W., McGrath, T. *et al.* (1984). A new *Legionella* species, *Legionella feeleii* species nova, causes Pontiac fever in an automobile plant. *Ann Intern Med* **100**, 333–8.

Holmes, R.L. (1982). Aniline blue-containing buffered charcoal yeast extract medium for presumptive identification of *Legionella* species. *J Clin Microbiol* **15**, 723–4.

Johnson, J.D., Raff, M. and Arsdall, J.A.V. (1984). Neurologic manifestations of Legionnaires' disease. *Medicine* **63**, 303–10.

Johnson, S.R., Schalla, W.O., Wong, K.H. and Perkins, G.H. (1982). Simple transparent medium for study of *Legionellae*. *J Clin Microbiol* **15**, 342–4.

Joly, J.R., McKinney, R.M., Tobin, J.O. *et al.* (1986). Development of a standardized subgrouping scheme for *Legionella pneumophila* serogroup 1 using monoclonal antibodies. *J Clin Microbiol* **23**, 768–71.

Joly, J.R. and Winn, W.C. (1984). Correlation of subtypes of *Legionella pneumo-*

phila defined by monoclonal antibodies with epidemiological classification of cases and environmental sources. *J Infect Dis* **150**, 667–71.

JAMA. 'Legionnaires' disease not limited to lungs'. (1980). **244**, 2597–601.

Kaan, J.A. and Maclaren, D.M. (1986). Comparison of media for recovery of Legionella pneumophila. *Am J Clin Pathol* **85**, 256–7.

Kalweit, W.H., Winn, W.C.. Rocco, T.A. and Girod, J.C. (1982). Haemodialysis fistula infections caused by Legionella pneumophila. Ann Intern Med **96**, 173–5.

Karr, D.E., Bibb, W.F. and Moss, C.W. (1982). Isoprenoid quinones of the genus *Legionella*. *J Clin Microbiol* **15**, 1044–8.

Keathley, J.D. and Winn, W.C. (1984). Comparison of media for recovery of *Legionella pneumophila* clinical isolates. In *Legionella: Proceedings of the 2nd International Symposium: Washington, DC.*, pp. 19–20. American Society for Microbiology, Washington.

Kerr, D.N.S., Brewis, R.A.L. and Macrae, A.D. (1978). Legionnaires' disease and acute rental failure. *Br Med J* **2**, 538–9.

Kohler, R.B., Zimmerman, S.E., Wilson, E. *et al.*, (1981). Rapid radioimmunoassay diagnosis of Legionnaires' disease. *Ann Intern Med* **94**, 601–5.

Kohne, D.E., Steigerwalt, A.G. and Brenner, D.J. (1984). Nucleic acid probe specific for members of the genus Legionella. In *Legionella: Proceedings of the 2nd International Symposium: Washington, DC.*, pp. 107–08. Edited by Thornsberry, C., Balows, A., Feeley, J.C. and Jakubowski, W. American Society for Microbiology, Washington.

Lancet (Editorial). (1983). Waterborne Legionella. **2**, 381–3.

Lees, A.W. and Tyrrell, W.F. (1978). Severe cerebral disturbance in Legionnaires' disease. *Lancet* **2**, 1336–7.

McDade, J.E., Shepard, C.C., Fraser, D.W. *et al.* (1977). Legionnaires' disease. Isolation of a bacterium and demonstration of its role in other respiratory disease. *N Engl J Med* **297**, 1197–203.

Macfarlane, J.T., Finch, R.G., Ward, M.J. and Macrae, A.D. (1982). Hospital study of adult community-acquired pneumonia. *Lancet* **2**, 255–8.

Macfarlane, J.T. and Ward, M.J. (1984). Transtracheal injection of saline in the investigation of pneumonia. *Br Med J* **288**, 974–5.

Matthay, R.A. and Moritz, E.D. (1981). Invasive procedures for diagnosing pulmonary infection. *Clin Chest Medicine* **2**, 3–18.

Moss, C.W., Bibb, W.F., Karr, D.E. *et al.* (1983). Cellular fatty acid composition and ubiquinone content of *Legionella feeleii* spp. nov. *J Clin Microbiol* **18**, 917–19.

Müller, H.E. (1981). Enzymatic profile of *Legionella pneumophila*. *J Clin Microbiol* **13**, 423–6.

Nelson, D.P., Rensimer, E.R. and Raffin, T.A. (1985). *Legionella pneumophila* pericarditis without pneumonia. *Arch Intern Med* **145**, 926.

Nolte, F.S., Hollick, G.E. and Robertson, R.G. (1982). Enzymic activities of *Legionella pneumophila* and *Legionella*-like organisms. *J Clin Microbiol* **15**, 175–7.

Orrison, L.H., Bibb, W.F., Cherry, W.B. and Thacker, L. (1983). Determination of antigenic relationships among legionella and non-legionellae by direct fluorescent antibody and immuno-diffusion tests. *J Clin Microbiol* **17**, 332–7.

Para, M.F. and Plouffe, J.F. (1983). Production of monoclonal antibodies to *Legionella pneumophila* serogroups 1 and 6. *J Clin Microbiol* **18**, 895–900.

Pasculle, A.W., Feeley, J.C., Gibson, R.J. *et al.* (1980). Pittsburgh pneumonia agent: direct isolation from lung tissue. *J Infect Dis* **141**, 727–32.

Pearson, S.B. and Dadds, J.H. (1981). Neurological complications of Legionnaires' disease. *Postgrad Med J* **57**, 109–10.

Rihs, J.D., Yu, V.L., Zuravleff, J.J. *et al.* (1985). Isolation of *Legionella pneumophila* from blood with the BACTEC system: a prospective study yielding positive results. *J Clin Microbiol* **22**, 422–4.

Rodgers, F.G. (1979). Ultrastructure of *Legionella pneumophila*. *J Clin Pathol* **32**, 1195–202.

Rodgers, F.G. (1983). The role of structure and invasiveness on the pathogenicity of Legionella. *Zbl Bakt Hyg I Abt Orig A* 1983; **255**, 138–44.

Rodgers, F.G. and Laverick, T. (1984). *Legionella pneumophila* serogroup 1 flagellar antigen in a passive haemagglutination test to detect antibodies to other *Legionella* species. In *Legionella: Proceedings of the 2nd International Symposium: Washington, DC.*, pp. 42–4. Edited by Thornsberry, C., Balows, A., Feeley, J.C. and Jakubowski, W. American Society for Microbiology, Washington.

Sathapatayavongs, B., Kohler, R.B., Wheat, J. *et al.* (1983). Rapid diagnosis of Legionnaires' disease by latex agglutination. *Am Rev Resp Dis* **127**, 559–62.

Schlanger, G., Lutwick, L.I., Kurzman, M. *et al.* (1984). Sinusitis caused by *Legionella pneumophila* in a patient with acquired immune deficiency syndrome. *Am J Med* **77**, 957–60.

Shaw, S., Dean, E. and Kohne, D. (1985). A rapid DNA probe for the specific detection of legionella species. *Abst Annu Meet Am Soc Microbiol*, 356.

Smith, M.G. (1982). A simple disc technique for the presumptive identification of *Legionella pneumophila*. *J Clin Pathol* **35**, 1353–5.

Strikas, R., Seifert, M.R. and Lentino, J.R. (1983). Autoimmune haemolytic anaemia and *Legionella pneumophila* pneumonia. *Ann Intern Med* **99**, 345.

Tang, P.W., de Savigny, D. and Toma, S. (1982). Detection of *Legionella* antigenuria by reverse passive agglutination. *J Clin Microbiol* **15**, 998–1000.

Tang, P.W., Toma, S., Moss, C.W. *et al.* (1984). *Legionella bozemanii* serogroup 2: a new etiological agent. *J Clin Microbiol* **19**, 30–33.

Taylor, A.G. and Harrison, T.G. (1981). Formolized yolk sac antigens in early diagnosis of Legionnaires' disease caused by *Legionella pneumophila* serogroup 1. *Lancet* **2**, 591–2.

Taylor, A.G. and Harrison, T.G. (1983). Serological tests for *Legionella pneumophila* serogroup 1 infections. *Zbl Bakt Hyg I Abt Orig A* **255**, 20–26.

Taylor, A.G., Harrison, T.G., Andrews, B.E. and Sillis, M. (1980). Serological differentiation of Legionnaires' disease and *Mycoplasma pneumoniae* pneumonia. *Lancet* **1**, 764.

Tenover, F.C., Carlson, L., Goldstein, L. *et al.* (1985). Confirmation of *Legionella pneumophila* cultures with a fluorescein-labelled monoclonal antibody. *J Clin Microbiol* **21**, 983–4.

Thacker, W.L., Plikaytis, B.B. and Wilkinson, H.W. (1985). Identification of 22 *Legionella* species and 33 serogroups with the slide agglutination test. *J Clin Microbiol* **21**, 779–82.

Vickers, R.M., Brown, A. and Garrity, G.M. (1981). Dye-containing buffered charcoal-yeast extract medium for the differentiation of members of the family Legionellaceae. *J Clin Microbiol* **13**, 380–82.

Wadowsky, R.M. and Yee, R.B. (1981). Glycine-containing selective medium for isolation of *Legionellaceae* from environmental specimens. *Appl Environm Microbiol* **42**, 768–72.

Wang, W.L.L., Blaser, M.J., Cravens, J. and Johnson, M.A. (1979). Growth, survival and resistance of the Legionnaires' disease bacterium. *Ann Intern Med* **90**, 614–18.

Watkins, I.D. and Tobin, J.O.H. (1984). Studies with monoclonal antibodies to *Legionella* species. In *Legionella: Proceedings of the 2nd International Symposium: Washington, DC.*, pp. 259–62. Edited by Thornsberry, C., Balows, A., Feeley, J.C. and Jakubowski, W. American Society for Microbiology, Washington.

Watkins, I.D., Tobin, J.O.H., Dennis, P.J. *et al.* (1985). *Legionella pneumophila* serogroup 1 subgrouping by monoclonal antibodies – an epidemiological tool. *J Hyg*, Camb **95**, 211–16.

Weaver, R.E. (1978). Cultural and staining characteristics: In *Legionnaires', the disease, the bacterium and methodology.*, pp. 18–21. Edited by Jones, G.L. and Hébert, G.A. CDC, Atlanta.

Wegmüller, E., Weidmann, P., Hess, T. and Reubi, F.C. (1985). Rapidly progressive glomerulonephritis accompanying Legionnaires' disease. *Arch Intern Med* **145**, 1711–13.

Weisenburger, D.D., Rappaport, H., Ahluwalia, M.S. *et al.* (1980). Legionnaires' disease. *Am J Med* **69**, 476–82.

Wilkinson, H.W. and Brake, B.J. (1982). Formalin-killed versus heat-killed *Legionella pneumophila* serogroup 1 antigen in the indirect immunofluorescence assay for legionellosis. *J Clin Microbiol* **16**, 979–81.

Wilkinson, H.W. and Fikes, B.J. (1980). Slide agglutination test for serogrouping *Legionella pneumophila* and atypical *Legionella*-like organisms. *J Clin Microbiol* **11**, 99–101.

Wilkinson, H.W., Cruce, D.D. and Broome, C.V. (1981). Validation of *Legionella pneumophila* indirect immunofluorescence assay with epidemic sera. *J Clin Microbiol* **13**, 139–46.

Wilkinson, H.W., Reingold, A.L., Brake, B.J. *et al.* (1983). Reactivity of serum from patients with suspected legionellosis against 29 antigens of Legionellaceae and legionella-like organisms by indirect immunofluorescence assay. *J Infect Dis* **147**, 23–31.

Winter, J.H., McCartney, A.C., Fallon, R.J. *et al.* (1986). Outbreak of Legionnaires' disease in Glasgow Royal Infirmary: early containment by rapid diagnosis. *Thorax* Abstract in press.

Wreghitt, T.G., Nagington, J. and Gray, J. (1982). An ELISA test for the detection of antibodies to *Legionella pneumophila*. *J Clin Pathol* **35**, 657–60.

Yee, R.B. and Wadowsky, R.M. (1982). Multiplication of *Legionella pneumophila* in unsterilized tap water. *Appl Environm Microbiol* **43**, 1330–34.

Yonke, C.A., Stiefel, H.E., Wilson, D.L. and Wentworth, B.B. (1981). Evaluation of an indirect hemagglutination test for *Legionella pneumophila* serogroups 1 to 4. *J Clin Microbiol* **13**, 1040–5.

Zuravleff, J.J., Yu, V.L., Shonnard, J.W. *et al.* (1983). Diagnosis of Legionnaires' disease. *JAMA* **250**, 1981–5.

7 Environmental Sources of Infection and Modes of Transmission

Sources of infection

Most cases of legionellosis have appeared to be sporadic and the source of these infections has been obscure. On the other hand the investigation of outbreaks of legionnaires' disease and Pontiac fever has led to the identification of several important sources of epidemic legionellosis. Although the initial outbreak which followed the American Legion convention in Philadelphia in 1976 was not fully explained, epidemiological studies suggested that airborne spread of legionella took place from an undetermined environmental reservoir. Subsequently, in other outbreaks cooling towers were soon recognized as sources; there was strong epidemiological evidence for this in a hospital outbreak (Dondero *et al.*, 1980) and in another associated with a hotel (Band *et al.*, 1981). Shortly afterwards piped water systems in hospitals (Fisher-Hoch *et al.*, 1981; Tobin *et al.*, 1980), and hotels (Tobin *et al.*, 1981) were implicated as further sources. Many other outbreaks from cooling towers and piped water distribution systems, particularly hot water circuits, in hotels and hospitals have now been documented. Clusters occurring in industrial and recreational settings have led to the recognition of other, less common, sources and vehicles of transmission. So far, the following have been shown to serve as sources of epidemic legionellosis:

Domestic hot water systems in large buildings.
Cooling water systems used for air-conditioning purposes.
Cooling water systems used for industrial purposes.
Spas/Whirlpools.
Industrial coolants used for grinding/machine lubrication.
  (88–99 per cent water and 1–12 per cent oil).
Respiratory therapy equipment.

In view of the widespread distribution of legionella species in aquatic habitats, it is tempting to speculate as to why other types of water systems, such as 'process' waters in industry have not been found to be sources. Furthermore, why should outbreaks of legionellosis occur only infrequently in association with hotels and hospitals, when most of these establishments, at least in Britain, harbour the organism (Bartlett *et al.*, 1986). To answer such questions it is helpful to consider a conceptual scheme of the chain of causation that leads from environmental site to infection in humans (Fraser, 1984):

(i)   That there exists an environmental reservoir where legionellas live.
(ii) That there be one or more amplifying factors which allow legionellas to grow from low to high concentration.
(iii) That there be a mechanism for dissemination of legionellas from the reservoir.
(iv) That the strain of legionella that is disseminated be virulent for humans.
(v)   That the organism be inoculated at an appropriate site on the human host.
(vi) That the host be susceptible to legionella infection.

Epidemiological studies of outbreaks have varied in the extent to which they have elucidated the various links in the chain, but successively they have built up a body of knowledge which has led to the development of effective control measures and suggested possibilities for primary prevention. Each of the sections below deal with the recognized sources of legionellosis, the outbreak investigations that substantially contributed to our understanding of the subject will be presented and the epidemiological evidence reviewed.

Domestic hot water systems in large buildings

Piped water systems have now been implicated as sources in many outbreaks associated with hospitals and hotels, some of which are described in Tables 7.1 and 7.2.

As there appears to be some variation internationally in the terms used to describe water distribution systems, Fig. 7.1 is included to illustrate the terminology applied by engineers in Britain and used in this chapter.

In all the outbreaks shown in Tables 7.1 and 7.2, legionellas of the same serogoup and species causing the outbreak were isolated also from the

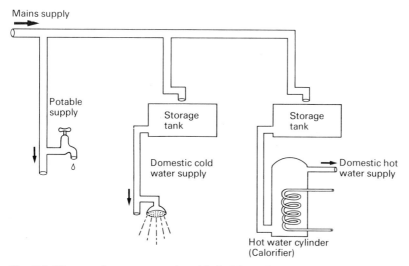

Fig. 7.1 Diagram of water systems in public buildings. From Bartlett, 1984.

Table 7.1 Outbreaks and case clusters from hospital domestic water systems*

Years	Place	Comments	Number of cases	Principal control measures
1975–80	Iowa, USA	Most cases associated with a newly opened 232 bedded unit, particularly haematology/oncology hospital	39	Shock and continuous chlorination ↑HW temperature temporarily
1977–80	Los Angeles, USA	Large cluster of cases followed a pressure 'shock' to the hospital domestic water systems	175 +	Continuous chlorination
1978–83	Leiden, Holland	A small cluster followed a fall in circulating HW temp	16	↑HW temperature
1979	Oxford, UK	—	2	Shock chlorination
1979–80	Melbourne, Australia	—	2	Shock chlorination
1979–80	Kingston, UK	A case that occurred after control measures coincided with a calorifier being brought on line	11	Continuous chlorination
1979–83	Pittsburgh, USA	—	26	↑HW temperature
1980–81	Pittsburgh, USA	Reduction in frequency of legionellosis after raising HW temperatures	100	↑HW temperature
1980–83	Cardiff, UK	Cases followed lowering of HW temperature	4	↑HW temperature
1981–84	Paris, France	3 patients occupied rooms served by one hot water pipe	4	
1982	Malone, USA	Water source was from a spring fed brook	6	Shock and continuous chlorination
1982	Rochester, USA	—	4	
1982–83	Columbus, USA		19	
1982–84	Pittsburgh, USA	(i) *L. bozemanii* isolated from adjacent excavation site	8	
1983–84	Stamford, USA	(ii) Pressure shock to hospital water system prior to outbreak	5	↑HW temperature

HW = Hot water

* Shown in chronological order rather than date of publication of paper

From Helms *et al.*, 1983; Shands *et al.*, 1985; Meenhorst *et al.*, 1985; Tobin *et al.*, 1980; Makela *et al.*, 1981; Fisher-Hoch *et al.*, 1981; Rudin *et al.*, 1984; Best *et al.*, 1983; Palmer *et al.*, 1986; Neill *et al.*, 1985; Stout *et al.*, 1982; Nolte *et al.*, 1984; Maher *et al.*, 1983; Johnson *et al.*, 1985; Parry *et al.*, 1985

Table 7.2 Outbreaks and case clusters from domestic water systems in hotels*

Years	Place	Water source	Comments	Number of cases	HW Temperature at outlets	Principal control measures
1973–80	Benidorm, Spain	Mains upland + own well with common cistern	(i) reintroduction of well supply. Preceeded outbreak in 1980 (ii) refrigeration unit cooling water (35°C) drained to the main cold water cistern	42 +	48°C	↑Hot water temperature continuous chlorination
1979	Corby, England	Mains (upland/river)	Flooding of plant room from underground stream preceded outbreak	5	44–48°C	↑Hot water temperature chlorination
1979–82	St. Croix, US Virgin Islands	Rain water/mains/well poured into two cisterns	–	15	not known	Shock chlorination
1980–82	Lido di Savio, Italy	Mains + own well with common cistern	Hotel closed during winter season	23	not known	Shock chlorination + well supply disconnected
1980–82	Quarteira, Portugal	Mains (borehole)	Solar heating system in hot water circuit	6	30.5–46°C	Solar heating disconnected
1980–83	Quarteira, Portugal	Mains (borehole)		14	22–58°C	Continuous chlorination

* Shown in chronological order rather than date of publication of paper
From Bartlett *et al.*, 1984; Reid *et al.*, 1978; Tobin *et al.*, 1981; Schlech *et al.*, 1985; Rosmini *et al.*, 1984; Bartlett and Bibby 1983

domestic hot water systems. Identical legionellas were recovered less frequently from the domestic cold water systems and only rarely from potable supplies. There has been no published account of an outbreak showing convincingly that an outbreak of legionellosis has resulted from a domestic cold water supply alone, so clearly temperature is one of the important amplification factors for legionellas which are virulent for man.

One of the major omissions in most of the papers from which Tables 7.1 and 7.2 were compiled was a record of circulating water temperatures. Hot water temperatures, recorded at taps after flushing are available for four of the hotel sites (see Table 7.2); minimum values range from 22–44°C. This suggests that the distribution of hot water at luke-warm temperatures may encourage multiplication and the absence of data on domestic hot water systems in hospitals associated with outbreaks is disappointing. Careful documentation of this and other aspects of engineering might shed some light on the temperatures and other factors to be avoided in water systems in large institutions. Most hospitals and many hotels in Britain now circulate hot water at temperatures in excess of 50°C. The dearth of information on other engineering aspects in the publications suggests that water and building services engineers have rarely been key members of outbreak investigation teams. Hopefully this oversight has now been recognized and its correction will be reflected in future publications.

Tobin and colleagues (1980) were the first to propose that 'interrupted' water supplies in hospitals could serve as sources of legionnaires' disease. They described two cases of *L. pneumophila* infection in patients who had recently had renal transplant surgery. Both had occupied the same single bedded cubicle, although there was an interval of 6 months between the two infections. *L. pneumophila* was isolated from bronchial aspirates from both patients and from the shower unit in the cubicle. All the isolates were of the same serogroup which was at first thought to be an atypical serogroup 3 and later shown to be serogroup 6. This serogroup is infrequently recovered from clinical or environmental specimens in the United Kingdom. Extensive sampling of other potential sources in the hospital, including the ventilation system, failed to detect this serogroup elsewhere. Powerful circumstantial evidence had, therefore, been produced to show that domestic water systems in hospitals were able to serve as a reservoir of legionella which could, at least, infect immunocompromised patients.

The findings of investigators in Oxford were soon substantiated in the investigation of a cluster of cases associated with a hotel in the English Midlands (Tobin *et al.*, 1981). This time it was shown not only that hotel domestic water systems could serve as sources but also that apparently immunocompetent individuals could be infected from them.

In the hotel-associated cluster, five cases of *L. pneumophila* serogroup 1 pneumonia and several pneumonias of unknown aetiology occurred within a month among guests. *L. pneumophila* serogroup 1 was recovered from hot and cold water storage tanks, taps and showers but from no other environmental samples collected in or around the hotel. Unlike the hospital in Oxford, the building did not have a ventilation system, and there was no air-conditioning system or cooling tower in its vicinity. Control measures were devised, somewhat empirically with continuous chlorination of the cold water supply to 1–2 mg/litre (ppm) and raising the hot water temperatures to at least 50°C as measured at outlets.

A further case of *L. pneumophila* serogroup 1 pneumonia occurred 2 years later in a man who became ill within a week of staying in one of the hotel rooms in which it had not been possible, for technical reasons, to achieve a minimum hot water temperature of 50°C (Bartlett and Bibby, 1983). *L. pneumophila* serogroup 1 was isolated from water taken from hot taps in the room, but not from samples collected from other parts of the hotel in which the circulating hot water had been maintained at the recommended 50–60°C. The hot water tap in the room in question was supplied by an exceptionally long spur or deadleg arising from the peripheral end of the circulating hot water loop. These findings suggested that the hot water system was the source of infection and furthermore that *L. pneumophila* might multiply in the peripheral parts of the systems.

The report of the findings in Oxford led Cordes and colleagues (1981a) in the USA, to evaluate the role of showers as possible disseminators at three sites where nosocomial legionnaires' disease had occurred. They found *L. pneumophila* of the same serogroups as had infected patients in the shower fittings in all three hospitals. They also recovered the organism more frequently from showers on wards associated with legionnaires' disease than those on wards in which cases had not been recognized.

Domestic water systems were again found to be responsible for two outbreaks of legionnaires' disease in Britain in 1980. Eleven cases occurred in association with one wing of Kingston-upon-Thames District General Hospital (Fisher-Hoch *et al.*, 1981). This building had a cooling tower on its roof but three patients acquired the infection before the cooling water system was brought into use for the summer season and four cases occurred after it was treated with twice weekly shock chlorination. The outbreak eventually terminated after the domestic cold water system was chlorinated to 1–2 mg/litre (ppm) free residual chlorine and the circulating hot water temperature raised to 50–55°C.

The second outbreak in 1980 occurred among British tourists who had stayed at a hotel in Benidorm, Spain. This hotel had been shown retrospectively (Reid, *et al.*, 1978) to have been associated with an outbreak of legionnaires' disease in 1973. As a result of national surveillance and other retrospective studies, cases of legionnaires' disease are now known to have occurred among guests staying at the hotel in eight of the years between its construction in 1971 and implementation of control measures in 1980 (Bartlett *et al.*, 1984). The investigation in 1980 found 59 cases of pneumonia, 23 diagnosed as legionnaires' disease, among guests who had stayed at the hotel that summer. Perhaps the unexplained pneumonias were due to legionella species or serogroups as yet unrecognized or perhaps may have been due to other unrelated organisms from the same environmental source. The hotel did not have a cooling tower but *L. pneumophila* was isolated from samples of the hotel's hot and cold water systems. The epidemiological investigation found that cases were more likely than controls to be the first to bathe or shower in the morning, suggesting again the multiplication of the organism in the peripheral parts of the plumbing. Two intriguing findings resulted from a review of engineering practices in the hotel.

First, it was discovered that the hotel normally supplemented the mains water supply with water from its own well. Because of a pump failure the well had been out of use for a month in the early summer. The first case of legionnaires' disease in the outbreak occurred within one week of the reconnection of the well supply. Perhaps *L. pneumophila* had grown to a high concentration in the stagnant water in the long length of pipe running from the well to the hotel's main tank and then this water had seeded the domestic water systems.

Second, it was discovered that as a water conservation measure, cooling water from the kitchen's refrigeration unit was piped back to the hotel's main cold water tank. The refrigeration unit's cooling water circuit may well have been a site of amplification of the organism. Unfortunately, chlorination had been undertaken shortly before the outbreak investigation began, so it was not possible to test this hypothesis. Continuous control measures were implemented, consisting of continuous chlorination of the domestic water systems to 1–3 mg/litre (ppm) free residual chlorine and raising hot water temperatures to 50–60°C as measured at the outlets.

No further cases have occurred in association with the Benidorm hotel, although it has been virtually fully occupied during the last four years and national surveillance has been maintained. In the hospital in Kingston-upon-Thames, however, a further nosocomial legionella infection occurred about 18 months after the introduction of similar control measures. A careful study of this case provided another important clue as to a reservoir and amplification site for legionella organisms (Fisher-Hoch, *et al.*, 1982). The patient had been an in-patient for a week having routine investigations then 3 days after discharge developed legionella pneumonia. A careful review of engineering practices in the hospital revealed that one of three calorifiers had been brought into operation while the patient was in hospital. This calorifier had been held in reserve in the summer months during which time it contained warm stagnant water. Nurses on the wards reported that the hot water supplies showed a brownish discolouration during the weeks following reconnection. *L. pneumophila* serogroup 1, the same serogroup as caused the infection, was isolated from this water. It was later discovered that the standby calorifier had been brought into use on the day the patient had a bath and shower. Examination of another standby calorifier found a thick brown liquid deposit at the bottom in which *L. pneumophila* serogroup 1 was found in high concentration.

It was concluded that calorifiers should be considered as potential sources of *L. pneumophila* and this has been confirmed by other investigators. A recent study in England in National Health Service hospitals (Bartlett *et al.*, 1986) found legionellas to be present in more than half the calorifiers studied, most of which were operating at the time of operation. Because the cold water 'make-up' to the calorifier generally feeds into its base (Fig. 7.1), a lukewarm zone is created in the lower part of the cylinder. Legionella was commonly found in the sediment or 'sludge', which collects in the base of the calorifier.

Another water engineering procedure appeared to precipitate a large outbreak of legionnaires' disease in a hospital in the USA in 1980 (Shands *et al.*, 1985). Nosocomial legionella infections began shortly after the Wadsworth

Memorial Hospital in Los Angeles was first occupied in early 1977. Between May 1977 and February 1980, nosocomial legionella infections occurred at a rate that averaged 4.5 cases per month from May 1977 to February 1980. A dramatic increase in number of legionnaires' disease cases was observed in March 1980 (Fig. 7.2). At the end of February the emergency water pump of the hospital had been tested by closing the valves from the hospital's main water storage tanks. The emergency pump had failed with a resultant rapid fall in pressure and a 'shock' effect throughout the system. The hospital water was described as black or brown for several weeks afterwards. A similar sequence of events was reproduced in an unoccupied wing of the hospital. A 30-fold increase in the concentration of *L. pneumophila* isolated from tap water samples was observed after the experimental pressure 'shock'. The hospital water supply was chlorinated continuously from July 1980 and a pronounced fall in the frequency of nosocomial legionnaires' disease was observed.

The link with hot water systems in hospitals was further strengthened by Meenhorst and colleagues (1985), who studied 21 cases of pneumonia which occurred in the Leiden University Hospital, Netherlands, between August 1978 and November 1983. The infections were caused by *L. pneumophila* serogroups 1 and 10, both of which were isolated from the domestic hot water system in the building in which 19 of the 21 patients had been admitted. Typing the *L. pneumophila* serogroup 1 strains by means of monoclonal antibodies showed that the patient and hot water isolates were identical. Furthermore, they had the same plasmid profiles.

The association between *L. pneumophila* nosocomial infections and colonized hot water systems was demonstrated fortuitously by Stout and colleagues (1982) in the USA. They began an extensive environmental survey for *L. pneumophila* in their hospital in Pittsburgh shortly before an outbreak of 14 culture confirmed cases of legionnaires' disease occurred. They found *L. pneumophila* to be present in water samples at all 10 sites studied immediately before the outbreak. Although there was no intervention, the number of sites yielding *L. pneumophila* decreased during the months following the outbreak.

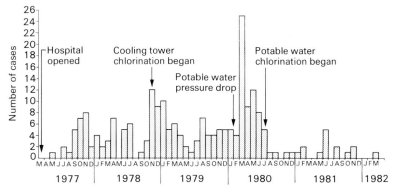

Fig. 7.2 Cases of legionnaires' disease, by month, at the Wadsworth Memorial Hospital, March 1977 through March 1982. There were no further cases in 1982 or 1983. From Shands *et al.*, 1985.

A further refinement to demonstrate the association was made by Johnson and colleagues (1985), who conducted a prospective study of pneumonia in two hospitals over 2 years. One hospital had a water supply contaminated with legionella, but no record of having had a case of legionnaires' disease, whereas the other had had its water supply decontaminated because of known endemic nosocomial legionellosis. Over the first 18 months, the rate of nosocomial legionellosis in high risk patients was 30 per cent at the first hospital and zero at the second. This study not only elegantly demonstrated a reservoir for nosocomial legionellosis but also drew attention to the fact that legionnaires' disease may be commonly missed, unless clinicians are actively considering the diagnosis.

Hot water systems in hospitals may also serve as a reservoir for legionella infections other than those due to *L. pneumophila*. Parry and colleagues (1985), studied five cases of nosocomial pneumonia due to *L. bozemanii*. Legionellas of the same species were isolated from four of the five infected patients, from tap water in the wards they occupied, from the hospital's hot water holding tanks, and from soil in an excavation area nearby. Chlorination and raising the hot water temperature eliminated *L. bozemanii* from the domestic water system and no further cases were detected. The significance of the isolation from soil is unclear, but it is possible that dust from the excavation site may have seeded the hospital water system. Best and colleagues (1983), investigated a nosocomial outbreak involving legionella pneumonias due to *L. pneumophila* and *L. micdadei*. Both species were isolated from the hospital's hot water system. Intermittent raising of the hot water temperature to 60–77°C produced a decline in the numbers of *L. pneumophila* and *L. micdadei* in the water system and was followed by a fall in the incidence of pneumonias from both species. Furthermore, a decrease both in the number of months in which nosocomial legionella infections occurred and the proportion of nosocomial pneumonias caused by these organisms was seen after the control measures were implemented. Muder and colleagues (1983), investigated seven patients with dual infections from *L. pneumophila* and *L. micdadei*. Both species were isolated from patients and the hospital's water system.

Together the results of the epidemiological investigations reviewed above or referred to in Tables 7.1 and 7.2 provide overwhelming evidence that domestic hot water systems in large buildings can serve as sources of legionellosis. Indeed, Johnson and colleagues (1985), have concluded that all five of Evans' modifications of Koch's postulates have been amply fulfilled (Evans, 1976). Each of the studies has shed light on at least one link in the chain of causation proposed by Fraser (1984). The demonstration of the reservoir is particularly convincing in the reports of the studies by Best and colleagues (1983), Johnson and colleagues (1985) and Meenhorst and colleagues (1985). Each showed a clear association between the presence of legionellas in the hot water system and the occurrence of legionellosis. In addition, several of the outbreak investigations can be considered as intervention studies (Bartlett, 1984). In each of the establishments shown in Table 7.3, control measures were applied to their domestic water supplies, particularly the hot water systems and these were followed by periods of extended surveillance for legionnaires' disease. Prior to the 'intervention',

Table 7.3 Intervention studies in establishments associated with legionnaires' disease *

| Place | Site | Cases in | Control measures began | Principal methods | Number of cases | |
					Before intervention	After intervention
Benidorm, Spain	Hotel	1973–80	1980	↑HW Temperature, chlorination	42+	0
Kingston, England	Hospital	1979–80	1980	↑HW Temperature, chlorination	11	2
Los Angeles, USA	Hospital	1977–80	1980	Chlorination	175+	6
Pittsburgh, USA	Hospital	1979–81	1981	↑HW Temperature	100+	12
Iowa City, USA	Hospital	1981	1981	Chlorination, ↑HW Temperature	24	0

HW = Hot water
* Shown in chronological order rather than date of publication of paper
   Data from references
   From Bartlett, 1984

legionnaires' disease had been shown to be associated with all but one of the establishments over a period of at least 2 years and, in one instance, 7 years (Bartlett *et al.*, 1984). No associated legionella infections have been detected since the intervention in two of the establishments, and dramatic falls in incidence have been reported in the other three. Later modifications of control measures in two of these three sites has virtually eliminated nosocomial legionella infection.

Amplification factors, other than temperature, in institutional domestic water systems have not been clearly defined although several studies have produced findings worthy of further investigation. The link with water temperature is quite impressive. Palmer and colleagues (1986), investigated a cluster of four cases of nosocomial legionnaires' disease in a hospital in Wales. A review of engineering procedures found that the domestic hot water had been maintained at a minimum of 60°C in the calorifier and 50°C at outlets. In July 1983, hot water temperatures were reduced by about 10°C in order to reduce working temperatures in the hospital's operating theatres. The cluster of cases occurred 2 months after this event during a 2 week period. Water collected from hot taps yielded *L. pneumophila* serogroup 1 which was indistinguishable by monoclonal antibody typing from isolates from two of the cases.

In Leiden, Meenhorst and colleagues (1985), identified two nosocomial legionella infections about 6 months after control measures were implemented in their hospital. It was found that the calorifier temperature had been accidentally lowered from 72°C to 52°C, resulting in temperatures within the range 36–49°C rather than about 60°C. The two cases occurred about a fortnight after this accident. Optimum temperatures to control the growth of legionella in hot water systems, yet not produce an unacceptable risk of scalding, have yet to be determined. Calorifiers seem to provide an ecological niche for legionellas (Fisher-Hoch, *et al.*, 1982). It is unclear whether the rust, scale and other debris which collect in the base of calorifiers provide a nutritional source for legionellas, or whether amplification may be explained solely by the ideal temperatures often found in the lower part of the cylinder. Stout and colleagues (1985) demonstrated that *L. pneumophila* could multiply actively in the sediment of hot water storage tanks and that the presence of other environmental bacteria acted synergistically to improve the survival of *L. pneumophila*.

Several incidents suggest the possibility of a factor which promotes the growth of the organism in the peripheral part of hot water systems.

(i)   A man developed legionnaires' disease after occupying a hotel room in which it had not been possible to raise the hot water temperature to a minimum of 50°C as recommended to control an earlier outbreak of legionnaires' disease in the building (Bartlett and Bibby, 1983).

(ii) Three patients in a hospital in France developed legionnaires' disease in the same 24 hour period, but although they were on different floors they were all in rooms supplied with hot water by one specific pipe of the eighteen hot water pipes supplying the patient areas (Neill *et al.*, 1985).

(iii) A case control study of the outbreak in 1980 in the hotel in Benidorm suggested that those who were first to bathe in the morning were more likely to acquire the infection (Bartlett *et al.*, 1984).

If, as these observations suggest, *L. pneumophila* can multiply in the ends of long runs of pipework or at outlets – are materials occasionally found there which will sustain growth of the bacterium? Colbourne and colleagues (1984), have suggested that some fittings such as rubber washers may fulfil this role. There is good evidence that such materials will encourage the growth of other organisms (Burman and Colbourne, 1976, 1979), so this suggestion certainly deserves further study.

Ciésielski and colleagues (1984), who studied the water system in a hospital following three nosocomial legionella infections, concluded that stagnation and tap (faucet) aerators favoured the growth of *L. pneumophila*. A review of the investigation of outbreaks from domestic water systems in hotels provides a pointer to another possible amplification factor (see Table 7.2). Remarkably, five of the six hotel sites were supplied with well water, in the sixth hotel (second in Table 7.2), the main water tank was located in a plant room which was frequently flooded with water from an underground stream. This apparent association with ground waters offers a clue that one or more chemical factors may be at work. A recent study (Bartlett *et al.*, 1986) suggests that the chloride content and electrical conductivity of waters warrants further study in this respect. The presence of organic compounds might also be worthy of further investigation.

The many epidemiological investigations of outbreaks of legionnaires' disease have failed to provide clear evidence on the mechanism for dissemination of legionellas from the reservoir in hot water systems to man. Case control studies have repeatedly been unable to show that cases bathed, showered or brushed their teeth more frequently than controls. The technical problem lies in the fact that most people appear to be immune to legionellas (Fraser, 1984), but no suitable test is available to identify the susceptibles from whom controls could be selected. Only a relatively small proportion of the population have circulating antibodies, so these do not provide a suitable means for discrimination. Fraser (1984), has recommended the development of an immunological method such as a skin test to permit clear separation of immune from susceptible people.

Despite these problems of study design, two investigations hinted at an epidemiological association with exposure to aerosols produced by running taps or showers. Hanrahan and colleagues (1984), showed that cases were significantly more likely than controls to have occupied beds which were closer to the hospital ward's shower facilities. They also found that the length of hospital stay was greater in cases than controls. They did not demonstrate that the association with proximity to showers was independent of this confounding effect, presumably because of small numbers. Isolates of *L. pneumophila* serogroup 1 from a patient and hot water samples were identical by monoclonal antibody sub-typing. This finding indicated that the hot water system was the reservoir of infection, but unfortunately, efforts to use their monitoring equipment to isolate the bacterium from aerosols in the vicinity of the showers were unsuccessful. In the investigation of the outbreak in the Benidorm hotel, Bartlett and colleagues (1984), demonstrated a link with bathing or showering and the development of legionnaires' disease but it must be borne in mind that the numbers studied were small. Despite the lack of firm epidemiological evidence, great emphasis has been placed on showers as disseminators of legionella although the role of water taps should not be overlooked.

Meenhorst and colleagues (1985), showed a link between the serogroup causing nosocomial legionellosis in their patients and the serogroup isolated from water samples taken from taps in the immediate vicinity of their patients. They reported that six of 21 patients were in protective isolation when they became infected and 12 patients, four of whom were completely confined to bed, had not showered in the hospital. The beds of these four patients were situated next to the taps in the ward. Fisher-Hoch and colleagues (1981a), were able to obtain bathing histories on eight of the eleven patients involved in the outbreak of legionnaires' disease in Kingston Hospital; none of the eight had showers but all had bathed in a conventional bath. Helms and colleagues (1983), who studied a nosocomial outbreak in the University of Iowa Hospital, found that five of eight cases took showers during their stay in hospital, but spent significantly less time showering than controls matched for age, sex and primary discharge diagnosis. The findings of these three groups of workers suggest that at least as much attention should be paid to hot water taps as showers when looking for potential disseminators of legionella.

L. pneumophila serogroup 1 may be found in most domestic water systems in large buildings, often in high concentration. If mechanisms for dissemination are also widespread then the infrequent occurrence of outbreaks of legionellosis may be explained by strain variation in virulence. A great deal of effort has been spent in the search for a virulence marker, but so far no well validated method has emerged. Several studies, however, have produced results which look promising. Plouffe and colleagues (1984), studied the plasmid profiles and monoclonal antibody reactivity of *L. pneumophila* serogroup 1 strains isolated from two hospital buildings. Both buildings had been colonized by similar numbers of this serogroup but 19 nosocomial cases of legionnaires' disease had occurred in one building and only one case in the other. Most strains isolated from the building associated with the outbreak contained no plasmids, whereas all those in the other building did. Fifteen of the 16 clinical strains and all the hot water strains in the first building agglutinated in the presence of a monoclonal antibody designated LP-1-81 (Para *et al.*, 1984). None of the environmental isolates or the remaining clinical strain from the patient in the other building were agglutinated by this antibody. They concluded that the surface antigen recognized by LP-1-81 may be important in determining the relative virulence of different *L. pneumophila* serogroup 1 strains.

Caution has to be exercised in the interpretation of these fascinating results because other undetermined factors in the chain of infection may have been absent in the building which remained free of epidemic legionellosis. Later experimental work, however, has shown virulence differences, at least for guinea-pigs, in the strains isolated from the two buildings (Bollin *et al.*, 1985).

Another monoclonal antibody typing scheme has led to the identification of *L. pneumophila* serogroup 1 sub-types which may be particularly virulent for humans (Watkins *et al.*, 1985). They studied clinical isolates from sporadic and epidemic infections and also a large number of environmental isolates from a variety of establishments, some of which were associated with legionella infections. They found that most of the clinical isolates fell into one of two sub-groups which they have designated Pontiac sub-group and Bellingham sub-group; these sub-groups were found only infrequently in environmental specimens.

Such findings should provide encouragement for other workers who are using alternative new technologies for the purpose of sub-typing and detection of virulence markers.

The investigation of outbreaks of legionnaires' disease from hot water systems has shed some light on sites of inoculation; these are reviewed in the Appendix which deals with routes of infection. Host susceptibility has been addressed in several case control studies and the identified risk factors are given in Chapter 3. Most people appear not to be susceptible to legionella infection (Fraser, 1984), but the factors responsible for this immunity remain obscure.

Cooling water systems used for air-conditioning purposes

Recirculating cooling water systems may be used to transfer heat from air-conditioning refrigeration units to the atmosphere. During operation, the cooling water is passed over condenser tubes which carry the hot refrigerant. The water, having taken up heat from the coils, is pumped to the top of a tower down which it is sprayed against a current of air (see Fig. 8.4). In this process heat is lost by evaporation. The function of an evaporative condenser is similar to that of a cooling tower, but instead of the refrigeration unit being located remotely the condenser coils are housed within the tower.

Large volumes of air are drawn through the cooling tower or evaporative condenser by means of one or more fans, and in the process take up water as vapour and droplets. The droplets in 'drift' from the tower are likely to contain organisms which are present in the circulating cooling water. Figure 7.3 shows the plume, consisting of the droplets or "drift" and water vapour, from a cooling tower on the roof of a hospital.

The first clue that cooling water systems could serve as sources of legionellosis was demonstrated in the retrospective investigation of an unexplained outbreak of 'flu-like' illness in 1968, now known as Pontiac fever (Glick *et al.*, 1978). Ninety-five of 100 employees in a health department building in Pontiac were affected in the explosive outbreak. Despite extensive laboratory studies, the aetiology remained obscure, although it was felt that a virus was unlikely to be responsible in view of an absence of secondary cases among family contacts. Following the first isolation of *L. pneumophila* in 1977, stored paired sera from cases were tested with an immunofluorescent antibody test and 32 persons had seronconversion or diagnostic rises against the legionella antigen. In 1968, the explosive onset of the epidemic, as well as lack of evidence supporting other modes of exposure, led the investigators to conclude that airborne spread of infection had taken place. Attention was focused on the air-conditioning system and it was found that when it was

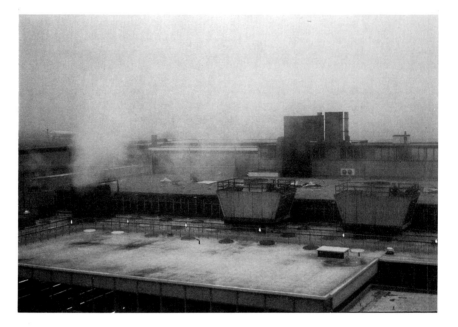

Fig. 7.3 Plume from a small capacity cooling tower in a hospital.

turned off one Saturday, persons newly exposed that day did not become ill within the observed incubation period range of 5–66 hours, but did become ill approximately 40 hours after entering the building the following Monday when the system was restarted. It was also found that attack rates were higher in persons entering the building on the Monday morning than in those first exposed that afternoon or evening, suggesting increased risk after restarting the air-conditioning system. Air was circulated within the building by means of metal ducting; the air intake was located on the roof top. An evaporative condenser for cooling purposes was situated in the basement of the building and there was a second ducting system to carry its exhaust to the roof top (Fig. 7.4). Smoke and gas tracer studies established that exhaust from the evaporative condenser could travel to the air inlets about 2 metres away and then be distributed around the building. Sentinel guinea-pigs which were placed in the building in 1968 developed pneumonia, but no aetiological agent was identified at that time. The frozen lung tissues were re-examined in 1977 and on this occasion *L. pneumophila* serogroup 1 was isolated. Identical strains were also recovered from guinea-pigs that had been exposed to aerosols of water taken from the evaporative condenser shortly after the outbreak. This impressive retrospective study showed, quite clearly, that the cooling water in the evaporative condenser was the source of the outbreak of Pontiac fever and that airborne transmission had taken place by means of the air-conditioning system.

Dondero and colleagues (1980), produced the earliest convincing evidence that cooling towers could also be responsible for legionnaires' disease in their

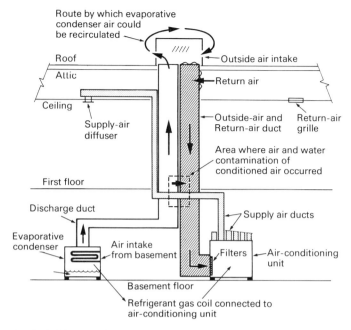

Fig. 7.4 Diagram of a cooling water system implicated in an outbreak of Pontiac fever. Adapted from Glick *et al.*, 1978.

report of an outbreak among patients, employees and visitors at a hospital in Memphis, USA in 1978. The onset of cases coincided with the use of an auxiliary cooling tower in the grounds of the hospital; the pumps for the main cooling towers had been inactivated by flooding following heavy rains. The first cases appeared within 3 days of the auxiliary cooling tower being turned on and the onset of the last case was 9 days after it was switched off (Fig. 7.5); the incubation period for legionnaires' disease ranges from 2–10 days (Fraser *et al.*, 1977). A case control study found that cases were significantly more

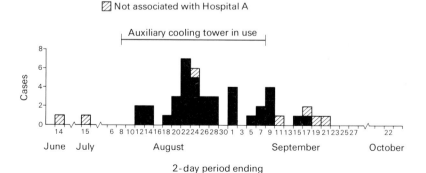

Fig. 7.5 Cases of legionnaires' disease by date of onset and by association with a hospital in Memphis (Hospital A). From Dondero *et al.*, 1980.

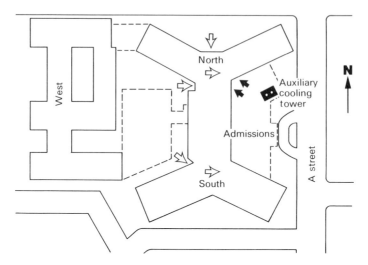

Fig. 7.6 Diagram of the hospital in Memphis. Black arrows indicate air intakes near cooling tower. White arrows indicate remote air intakes. From Dondero *et al.*, 1980.

likely than controls to have occupied rooms in the North wing of the hospital that were ventilated with air taken from near the cooling tower (Fig. 7.6).

Smoke tracer studies showed that drift from the tower could easily reach the ventilation system air intakes, as well as the street below where four passers-by had been before they contracted legionnaires' disease. *L. pneumophila* serogroup 1, the serogroup responsible for the outbreak, was isolated from water samples taken from the tower. This auxiliary unit, which had not been operated for nearly 2 years prior to the outbreak, had inadvertently not received chemical treatment of its water.

In July 1978, an outbreak of legionnaires' disease occurred among golfing members of a country club in Atlanta, USA (Cordes *et al.*, 1980). Those affected played significantly more holes of golf than control golfers during the likely time of exposure. There appeared to be a continuing source of infection in that no one day was identified on which all eight persons developing legionnaires' disease attended the club or played golf. *L. pneumophila* serogroup 1 was isolated from an evaporative condenser, the exhaust duct from which was directed towards a nearby practice green and the 10th and 16th tees (Fig. 7.7). It was concluded that the outbreak resulted from airborne dissemination from the evaporative condenser to adjacent parts of the golf course where susceptible golfers contracted the illness.

An investigation of an outbreak of legionnaires' disease in 1979 in Eau Claire, USA, found that a cooling tower on the roof of a hotel complex was the source of infection (Band *et al.*, 1981). Furthermore, it was shown that the drift from the cooling tower was carried to a meeting room, where the infections were probably contracted, by means of a chimney stack and disused fireplace. The visitors who had developed legionnaires' disease visited the part of the hotel that contains its restaurants and meeting rooms. Legionnaires' disease was identified in 1 per cent of those who had only been

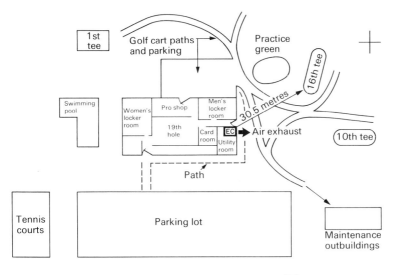

EC Evaporative condenser

Fig. 7.7 Location of evaporative condenser at a country club in Atlanta, Georgia, 1978. From Cordes *et al.*, 1980.

in the meeting rooms and in 0.1 per cent in those who had entered the restaurants. The highest attack rate of 1.5 per cent was found in those who had visited the meeting room with the fireplace. *L. pneumophila* serogroup 1, the causative agent, was isolated from the roof top cooling tower. Tracer studies with smoke and oil of wintergreen, demonstrated the retrograde flow of cooling tower exhaust down the chimney and into the meeting room. The outbreak stopped following the sealing of the chimney and treatment of the cooling water system by continuous chlorination.

Several other outbreaks from cooling water systems have been well documented. In one incident, a cooling tower probably served as a source of legionella infection over a 4-year period, with major outbreaks in 1977 and 1980 (Klaucke *et al.*, 1984). In both outbreaks, both nosocomial and community acquired infections were identified. Cases who had not visited the hospital during the 10 days before onset were mostly in individuals with residences down wind of the cooling tower which was located on a roof of a university building. *L. pneumophila* serogroup 1 isolates were identical by monoclonal antibody typing to strains isolated from patients during both outbreaks (Joly and Winn, 1984). This strong circumstantial evidence indicates that the tower was the source of the nosocomial and community acquired infections. The tower was located 150 metres away from the hospital building, indicating that *L. pneumophila* will survive in aerosol over a long distance under suitable ambient conditions.

The cause of a large nosocomial outbreak in Stafford, UK in 1985 was traced to a cooling tower on the roof of the hospital (Committee of Inquiry, 1986; O'Mahony *et al.*, 1986). *L. pneumophila* serogroup 1 isolated from the cooling water was identical to clinical isolates by monoclonal antibody subtyping. Inspection of the air-conditioning system showed that there was a direct communication between the ventilation system and the drain stack down which cooling water was discharged to waste. The communication existed because a drain from a condensate tray in the duct work passed directly to the same waste stack without a customary air break. Retrograde flow of cooling water into the ventilation system was found to take place when the building services were carefully inspected. In addition, *L. pneumophila* serogroup 1 of the same monoclonal antibody sub-group as clinical and cooling water isolates was recovered from this part of the ventilation system. Studies are still underway to determine whether entry of cooling water in this fashion, or as drift being drawn into the inlet for the ventilation system, was the principal mechanism for aerosol contamination of the conditioned air. A Committee of Inquiry (1986) concluded that the drift drawn into the inlet was the main way in which the organism was disseminated. O'Mahony and colleagues (1986) consider that this theory is not supported by the available epidemiological evidence.

Together these outbreak studies have shown conclusively that cooling waters serve as reservoirs of legionella infection and that cooling towers and evaporative condensers may effectively disseminate the organism. They have not, however, shed much light on amplification mechanisms and further studies are needed to elucidate these.

It is conventional practice to treat cooling water systems with scale and corrosion inhibitors and biocides to minimize organic fouling and thus maintain the efficiency of heat exchange. Few of the reports commented on the adequacy or indeed the existence of such treatment programmes for the implicated cooling waters. Several reports, however, stated clearly that there had been no treatment prior to the outbreak. Apart from lack of treatment, or inadequate treatment with biocides, stagnation may have been a contributory factor; in several instances outbreaks appeared to have followed periods when the cooling water systems were temporarily out of operation.

Non-pneumonic legionellosis (Pontiac fever) from cooling water systems was clearly demonstrated and in some outbreaks (Table 7.4), cases of both Pontiac fever and legionnaires' disease were identified. In one incident, two maintenance workers cleaned the interior of a cooling tower and subsequently developed legionellosis (Girod *et al.*, 1982). One man who entered the cooling tower when the fans were still in operation went on to develop legionnaires' disease. His colleague, who entered the tower several minutes after the fans were turned off, subsequently developed Pontiac fever. It is unclear why there should be two distinct clinical presentations of legionellosis. In this incident both men were likely to have been exposed to viable organisms although there may well have been differences in inoculum size or the particle sizes to which they had been exposed. There may also have been differences in host defence mechanisms and the relative contribution of these factors remains open to speculation.

Cooling water systems used for industrial purposes

Cooling water systems are widely used in industry, particularly in power generation and chemical processing. It is important to emphasize that the

Table 7.4 Outbreaks from cooling towers or evaporative condensers*

Years	Place	Source	Comments	Clinical presentation	Number of cases	Tower – chemically treated prior to outbreak	Control measure
1968	Pontiac, USA	Evaporative condenser in a health department building	Transmission by means of a defective air-conditioning system to staff and visitors	P.F.	144	Not known	Evaporative condenser relocated
1973	James River, USA	Steam turbine condenser	All cases took part in routine cleaning of the condenser	P.F.	10		
1977–80	Burlington, USA	Cooling tower (150 m from a hospital) on the roof of a university building	Community and hospital acquired cases associated with this tower	L.D.	85+	Intermittent chlorination only	Tower dismantled
1978	Atlanta, USA	Evaporative condenser located in a golf clubhouse	A case control study found the degree of golfing activity to be a risk factor – aerosol blown across the greens	L.D.	8	Once monthly only	Chlorination
1978	Memphis, USA	Auxiliary cooling tower in the grounds of a hospital	Cases were associated with exposure to vicinity of tower and parts of hospital ventilation with air drawn from near the tower	L.D.	44	No	Tower taken cut of use
1979	Eau Claire, USA	Cooling tower on the roof of a hotel	Airborne transmission from tower to persons in a meeting room by means of a chimney stack	L.D.	13	No	Tower treated with chlorination and followed by quarterly ammonium compound

Table 7.4 *Continued*

Years	Place	Source	Comments	†Clinical presentation	Number of cases	Tower – chemically treated prior to outbreak	Control measure
1979	Vasteras, Sweden	Cooling tower on the roof of indoor shopping centre	–	L.D.	58	Not known	Not known
1980	San Francisco, USA	Cooling tower on the roof of a new office building	Outbreak among office staff was temporary, associated with the use of the cooling tower	L.D. and P.F.	14	Not known	Shock chlorination
1980	Burlington, USA	Cooling tower on roof	Two men contracted legionellosis while cleaning interior of the tower	L.D. P.F.	2	Not known	Shock chlorination
1981	Rhode Island, USA	Cooling towers in the grounds and on the roof of a hospital building	Airborne transmission through open windows from tower 30 m away	L.D.	15	Yes; with a QUAT	Shock chlorination
1981	Heysham, UK	Compressor unit cooling towers in a power station under construction	Cases worked in vicinity of tower or in an adjacent building	L.D. P.F.	6	No	Chlorinated phenolic thio ether
1984	Glasgow, UK	Cooling tower 10 m above ground level	Most cases lived downwind of the tower	L.D.	33	Not known	Chlorination and chlorinated thioether
1985	Stafford, UK	Cooling tower on a hospital roof	Tower drift was shown to enter hospital ventilation system but a direct communication was also found between cooling tower drain and the ventilation system	L.D.	68	Yes	Shock and continuous chlorination. Direct link between drain and ventilation system broken
1985	Glasgow, UK	Cooling tower on a hospital roof	–	L.D.	16	Not known	Shock chlorination

* Shown in chronological order rather than date of publication of paper
Data from references

† L.D. = Legionnaires' disease
 P.F. = Pontiac fever

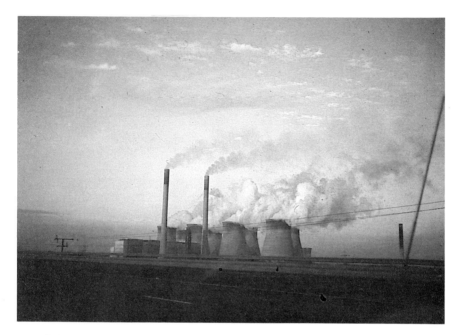

Fig. 7.8 Large scale natural updraft cooling towers used in industry. Such towers have never been found to be the source of an outbreak of legionnaires' disease.

large scale natural updraft cooling towers (Fig. 7.8) found in these industries have never been implicated as sources of legionellosis among those visiting or living in their vicinity. However, there is one instance of an outbreak of Pontiac fever occurring in men who had cleaned a steam turbine condenser on a power station (Fraser *et al.*, 1979). The incident occurred in Virginia, USA in 1973 and was recognized retrospectively as legionellosis through the examination of stored serum specimens. Ten previously fit men spent 9 hours working inside the condenser and subsequently all developed a severe, flu-like illness. The method of cleaning was to remove slime and debris by means of blasts of compressed air. It is likely that a dense aerosol from the slime materials was produced as a result of this procedure. It was reported that the temperature of the cooling water at the end of the cooling cycle was approximately 36°C at the time of the outbreak. Before being cleaned, the turbine had been allowed to cool for 2 days but had not been treated with chemicals. This study clearly identified the occupational risk associated with cleaning untreated cooling water systems by air blasting.

Another outbreak of legionellosis was recognized in an industrial setting in Heysham, UK in 1981. Six men working in a power station under construction developed legionnaires' disease during a 1 month period in the early autumn; another man developed Pontiac fever at the same time. A case control study found an association with working in the vicinity of, or in the building adjacent to, a battery of small capacity cooling water systems (Morton *et al.*, 1986). *L. pneumophila* serogroup 1 was isolated from the cooling waters, but from none of the numerous other environmental specimens that were collected on the site. The cooling waters had not received

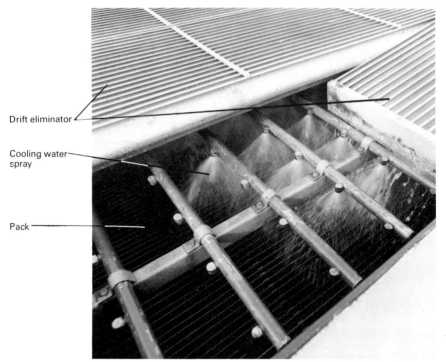

Fig. 7.9 Illustration of a cooling tower with drift eliminator partially removed to show the cooling water being sprayed over the pack.

conventional chemical treatment at any time prior to the outbreak. Further-more, a drift eliminator (Fig. 7.9) on the top of one had completely collapsed and fallen into the base of the tower. Another factor which may have led to the outbreak was the pattern of use of the equipment. The cooling systems were used intensively while the compressors were in use, then a period of several days or even weeks would elapse before they were operated again. This stagnation may have contributed to the multiplication of *L. pneumophila* in the cooling water.

Whirlpools and spas

Whirlpools, whirlpool spas and spas are recreational pools. The terms are often used interchangeably, although those involved in the industry use them quite specifically. A spa is a bath designed for sitting rather than swimming, and the water is filtered and chemically treated but usually not drained, cleaned or refilled after each user. They are of variable size, but commonly are designed to seat four to six persons. Spas are usually heated to about 37°C and often have air and water jets to produce turbulence. Strictly speaking, a whirlpool is a bath which is drained and cleaned after each user and often is not filtered or chemically treated. Like spas, they are often fitted with air and water jets. The generic term whirlpool spa is now coming into popular use, probably because it differentiates between the traditional health spa and the recreational pool.

The first documented outbreak of legionellosis from a whirlpool spa occurred in Vermont, USA in 1981 (Spitalny *et al.*, 1984). Altogether 34 of 74 members of a social club who visited an inn in a skiing resort developed Pontiac fever. A serological survey of members of the social club found that symptoms were significantly related to higher geometric mean titres to *L. pneumophila* serogroup 6 and *L. dumoffii*, but not to *L. pneumophila* serogroups 1 to 4. A highly significant association was found between development of symptoms and use of the whirlpool spa. *L. pneumophila* serogroup 1, serogroup 6 and *L. dumoffii* were isolated from the whirlpool water. Other samples taken from the inn including samples from the hot and cold domestic water systems, swimming pool and dehumidifiers were all negative for legionellas. Spitalny and colleagues (1984), concluded that two factors may have enhanced transmission of legionella by the whirlpool spa: first, there may have been inadequate chlorination of the pool water; and second, there was inadequate ventilation in the spa room. There were only two small exhaust fans to move air from the spa room to the outside of the building and there were no fresh air intakes, or windows nearby. The only entrance to the room was a single sliding glass door.

Another outbreak of Pontiac fever from a whirlpool spa was detected in Rochester, USA in 1982. Members of a church group attended an evening raquetball party and, within the next 48 hours, 14 of the 47 participants developed Pontiac fever (Mangione *et al.*, 1985). All 14 were women who had used a whirlpool spa in the women's locker room. Nine other women and all 24 men who had attended the party had not used the whirlpool spa and remained well. *L. pneumophila* serogroup 6 was isolated from the whirlpool spa water and this serogroup was shown by serology to be responsible for the outbreak. On this occasion aerosol size studies were undertaken and these showed that the whirlpool spa produced water droplets from 2–8 μ in size which are small enough to travel deep into the trachiobronchial tree, yet large enough to transport *L. pneumophila*.

The first outbreak of legionnaires' disease from whirlpool spas was recognized among guests who had visited a hotel in Brighton, UK in the early summer of 1984 (Public Health Laboratory Service, 1985). Twenty-six cases of pneumonia were found in association with the hotel, 16 of whom were shown to be legionnaires' disease. *L. pneumophila* serogroup 1, the serogroup responsible for the outbreak, was isolated from hot and cold domestic water systems in the hotel and from two whirlpool spas. A case control study demonstrated a strong association with use of the whirlpool spas and acquisition of legionnaires' disease. The whirlpool spas had been poorly maintained and a log of water treatment and test results were not kept. During the period prior to the outbreak, the only chemical treatment had consisted of once daily manual dosing with sodium hypochlorite solution to achieve an initial level of 5 mg/litre of free residual chlorine. This is likely to have persisted for a transient period only and indeed no free residual chlorine was detected at the time the pools were sampled; the temperature in one whirlpool spa was 36°C and the other 35°C. The filters in both whirlpool spas were found to be clogged with hair and other debris. Inadequate maintenance was obviously an important factor; the question of the chemical treatment of spas and whirlpools will be considered in Chapter 8.

Industrial coolants used for grinding machine lubrication

In August 1981, 317 workers in a car assembly plant developed Pontiac fever (Herwaldt *et al.*, 1984). A new legionella species, *Legionella feeleii*, was isolated from cooling fluids in the plant. The coolant systems lubricated, cooled and cleaned grinding machines surfaces. The coolant fluids used, consisted of 88–99 per cent water and 1–12 per cent oil. Caustics were added, as needed, to keep the coolants' pH between 8.5 and 9.5; biocides were added when the bacterial count exceeded 10^5 organisms/millilitre. Geometric mean titres against *L. feeleii* were significantly higher in those with Pontiac fever compared with controls. The proportion of workers affected in a department decreased linearly with the distance of the working area from the implicated coolant system. Smoke candle studies in the assembly plant suggested that coolant aerosols could be spread over a large area in relatively high concentrations. It may be significant that the coolant system which was found to be the source was shut down for 1 week prior to the outbreak but brought back into use shortly before the first cases presented. The investigators put forward the hypothesis that during the period of disuse bacterial overgrowth, which is known to occur more rapidly when coolants are not circulated, decreased the pH of the coolant and led to separation of the oil-water emulsion. This separation could have favoured the growth of *L. feeleii*.

Respiratory therapy equipment

The retrospective investigation of five cases of nosocomial legionnaires' disease in a hospital in Chicago in 1980 (Arnow *et al.*, 1982) lead to the recognition of respiratory therapy equipment as possible sources of the infection. All five patients during the 2–10 day period before onset of illness had either inhaled aerosolized tap water from jet nebulizers or from a portable room humidifier, and all had received high doses of corticosteroids or adrenocorticotrophic hormone. A highly significant difference in exposure to these factors was found when comparing cases with control patients. *L. pneumophila* was isolated from tap water and from water collected from the reservoirs in the respiratory therapy devices. This study did not show conclusively that the respiratory therapy equipment was the source of infection but obviously the use of tap water in such devices may well represent a hazard for patients who are immunocompromised. Although no other workers have substantiated the findings of Arnow and colleagues (1982), another single case probably from a mechanical humidifier has been reported from the Netherlands (Kaan *et al.*, 1985). A 64-year old man developed pneumonia after laryngectomy for a supraglottic squamous cell tumour. The man's room had been humidified by means of a small mechanical humidification device. The reservoir of the humidifier was refilled from a jerrycan which contained demineralized water. *L. pneumophila* serogroup 1 was isolated from this jerrycan. The strain appeared to be identical by sub-typing to an isolate which was made from material obtained from the patient at bronchoscopy. A similar strain was also isolated from the hot water system in the hospital, so it is possible that either reservoir may have been the source of infection. Kaan and colleagues (1985), however, concluded that the humidifier was the most likely source and banned the use of these devices in the hospital.

There is also some experimental evidence to show that small mechanical humidifiers might serve as sources of legionellosis. Zuravleff and colleagues (1983), collected water samples from the reservoir of another type of room humidifier and found them to be contaminated with *L. pneumophila*. Exposure of culture mediums to aerosols generated by the humidifier yielded *L. pneumophila* serogroup 1, and guinea-pigs that were exposed produced subclinical infections demonstrated by seroconversion to *L. pneumophila*. Gorman and colleagues (1980) isolated *L. micdadei* from nebulisers although associated disease was not reported. These reports indicate a potential risk from the use of tap water in room humidification devices and nebulizers in the management of patients with respiratory problems, particularly those who are immunocompromised.

Other potential sources and routes of infection (see Appendix)

References

Ad-Hoc Committee. (1986). Outbreak of legionellosis in a community report of an Ad-Hoc Committee. *Lancet* ii, 380–3.

Arnow, P.M., Chou, T., Weil, D. *et al.* (1982). Nosocomial Legionnaires' disease caused by aerosolized tap water from respiratory devices. *J Infect Dis* **146**, 460–67.

Band, J.D., LaVenture, M., Davis, J.P. *et al.* (1981). Epidemic Legionnaires' disease; airborne transmission down a chimney. *JAMA* **245**, 2404–7.

Bartlett, C.L.R. (1984). Potable Water as Reservoir and Means of Transmission. In *Legionella. Proceedings of the 2nd International Symposium Washington, DC.*, pp. 210–15. Edited by Thornsberry, C., Balows, A., Feeley J.C. and Jakubowski, W.J. American Society for Microbiology, Washington.

Bartlett, C.L.R. and Bibby, L.F. (1983). Epidemic Legionellosis in England and Wales 1979–1982. *Zentralblatt fur Bakteriologie, Parasitenkunde, Infektionskrankheiten und Hygiene I. Abteilung: Originale* A **255**, 64–70.

Bartlett, C.L.R., Dennis, P.J.L., Harper, D. *et al.* (1986). Legionella in plumbing systems. Submitted for publication.

Bartlett, C.L.R. and Pickering, C.A.C. (1983). Medical aspects of air conditioning and other building services. In *Air Conditioning System Design for Building.* Edited by A.F.C. Sherratt, McGraw Hill, London.

Bartlett, C.L.R., Swann, R.A., Canada Royo, C.L. *et al.* (1984). Recurrent Legionnaires' disease from a hotel water system. In *Legionella. Proceedings of the 2nd International Symposium: Washington, DC.*, pp. 237–9. Edited by Thornsberry, C., Balows, A., Feeley, J.C. and Jakubowski, W.J. American Society for Microbiology, Washington.

Baskerville, A., Broster, M., Fitzgeorge, R.B., *et al.* (1981). Experimental transmission of Legionnaires' disease by exposure to aerosols of legionella pneumophila. *Lancet* ii, 1389–90.

Best, M., Stout, J., Muder, R.R. *et al.* (1983). Legionellaceae in the hospital water supply. *Lancet* ii, 307–10.

Bollin, G.E., Plouffe, J.F., Para, M.F. *et al.* (1985). Difference in virulence of environmental isolates of *Legionella pneumophila*. *J Clin Microbiol* 21, 674–7.

Burman, N.P., Colbourne J.S. (1976). The effect of plumbing materials on water quality. *J Inst Plumb* 3, 13.

Burman, N.P., Colbourne J.S. (1979). Effect of non-metallic materials on water quality. *J Inst Water Eng Sci* 1, 11–18.

Ciesielski, C.A., Blaser, M.J., Laforce, M. *et al.* (1984). Role of stagnation and obstruction of water flow in isolation of *Legionella pneumophila* from hospital plumbing. In *Legionella. Proceedings of the 2nd International Symposium: Washington, DC.*, pp. 307–9. Edited by Thornsberry, C., Balows, A., Feeley, J.C. and Jakubowski, W.J. Am Soc Microbiol, Washington.

Colbourne, J.S., Pratt, D.J., Smith, M.G. *et al.* (1984). The role of water fittings as sources of *Legionella pneumophila* in a hospital's plumbing system. *Lancet* i, 210–13.

Committee of Inquiry (1986). First report of the Committee of Inquiry into the Outbreak of Legionnaires' disease in Stafford in April, 1985, London p. 22. HMSO, London.

Conwill, D.E., Benson Werner, S., Dritz, S.K. *et al.* (1982). Legionellosis, the 1980 San Francisco outbreak. *Am Rev Infect Dis* 126, 666–9.

Cordes, L.G., Fraser, D.W., Skaliy, P. *et al.* (1980). Legionnaires' disease outbreak in an Atlanta, Georgia, Country Club: evidence for spread from an evaporative condenser. *Am J Epidemiol* 111, 425–31.

Cordes, L.G., Wiesenthal, A.M., Gorman, G.W. *et al.* (1981). Isolation of *Legionella pneumophila* from Hospital Shower Heads. *Ann. Intern. Med* 94, 195–7.

Dondero, T.J., Rendtorff, R.C., Mallison, G.F. *et al.* (1980). An outbreak of Legionnaires' disease associated with a contaminated air-conditioning cooling tower. *N Engl J Med* 302, 365–70.

Evans, A. (1976). Causation and disease. The Henle-Koch postulates revised. *Yale J Biol Med* 49, 175–9.

Fisher-Hoch, S.P., Bartlett, C.L.R., and Harper, G.J. (1981a). Legionnaires' disease at Kingston Hospital. *Lancet* i, 1154.

Fisher-Hoch, S.P., Smith, M.G., Colbourne, J.S. (1982). *Legionella pneumophila* in hospital hot water cylinders. *Lancet* i, 1073.

Fisher-Hoch, S.P., Tobin, J.O'H., Nelson, A.M. *et al.* (1981b). Investigation and control of an outbreak of Legionnaires' disease in a District General Hospital. *Lancet* i, 932–6.

Fraser, D.W., Deuber, D.C., Hill, D.L. *et al.* (1979). Nonpneumonic, short-incubation-period legionellosis (Pontiac fever) in men who cleaned a steam turbine condenser. *Science* 205, 690–91.

Fraser, D.W. (1984). Sources of Legionellosis. In *Legionella. Proceedings of the 2nd International Symposium: Washington, D.C.*, pp. 277–80. Edited by Thornsberry, C., Balows, A., Feeley, J.C. and Jakubowski, W.J. American Society for Microbiology, Washington.

Fraser, D.W., Tsai, T.R., Orenstein, W. *et al.* (1977). Legionnaires' disease: description of an epidemic of pneumonia. *N Engl J Med* 297, 1189–97.

Garbe, P.L., Davis, B.J., Weisfeld, J.S. *et al.* (1985). Nosocomial Legionnaires' disease: Epidemiologic demonstration of cooling towers as a source. *JAMA* 254, 521–4.

Girod, J.C., Reichman, R.C., Winn, W.C. *et al.* (1982). Pneumonic and nonpneumonic forms of legionellosis. The result of a common-source exposure to *Legionella pneumophila. Arch Intern med* **142**, 545–7.

Glick, T.H., Gregg, M.B., Berman, B. *et al.* (1978). Pontiac fever: an epidemic of unknown etiology in a health department: I. clinical and epidemiologic aspects. *Am J Epidemiol* **107**, 149–60.

Gorman, G.W., Yu, V.L., Brown, A. *et al.* (1980). Isolation of Pittsburgh pneumonia agent from nebulizers used in respiratory therapy. *Ann Intern Med* **93**, 572–3.

Haley, C.E., Cohen, M.L., Halter, J., *et al.* (1979). Nosocomial Legionnaires' disease: A continuing common-source epidemic at Wadsworth Medical Center. *Ann Intern Med* **90**, 583–6.

Hanrahan, J.P., Morse, D.L., Scharf, V.B. *et al.* (1984). Community Hospital legionellosis outbreak linked to hot water showers. In *Legionella. Proceedings of the 2nd International Symposium: Washington, DC.*, pp. 224–5. Edited by Thornsberry, C., Balows, A., Feeley, J.C. and Jakubowski, W.J. Am Soc Microbiol, Washington.

Helms, C.M., Massanari, R.M., Zeitler, R. *et al.* (1983). Legionnaires' disease associated with a hospital water system: A cluster of 24 nosocomial cases. *Ann Intern Med* **99**, 172–8.

Herwaldt, L.A., Gorman, G.W, McGrath, T. *et al.* (1984). A new Legionella species, *Legionella feeleii* species nova, causes Pontiac fever in an automobile plant. *Ann Intern Med* **100**, 333–8.

Johnson, J.T., Best, M.G., Goetz, A. *et al.* (1985). Nosocomial legionellosis in surgical patients with head and neck cancer: implications for epidemiological reservoir and mode of transmission. *Lancet* **ii**, 298–300.

Joly, J.R. and Winn, W.C. (1984). Correlation of subtypes of *Legionella pneumophila* defined by monoclonal antibodies with epidemiological classification of cases and environmental sources. *J Infect Dis* **150**, 667–71.

Kaan, J.A., Simoons-Smit, A.M. and MacLaren, D.M. (1985). Another source of aerosol causing nosocomial legionnaires' disease. *J Infect* **11**, 145–8.

Klaucke, D.N., Vogt, R.L., LaRue, D. *et al* (1984). Legionnaires' disease: The epidemiology of two outbreaks in Burlington, Vermont 1980. *Am J Epidemiol* **119**, 382–91.

Maher, W.E., Plouffe, J.F. and Para, M.F. (1983). Plasmid profiles of clinical and environmental isolates of *Legionella pneumophila* serogroup 1. *J Clin Microbiol* **18**, 1422–3.

Makela, T.M., Harders, S.J., Cavanagh, P., *et al.* (1981). Isolation of *Legionella pneumophila* (serogroup 1) from shower-water in Ballarat. *Med J Austr* **1**, 293–4.

Mangione, E.J., Remis, R.S., Tait, K.A. *et al.* (1985). An outbreak of Pontiac fever related to whirlpool use, Michigan 1982. *JAMA* **253**, 535–9.

Meenhorst, P.L., Reingold, A.L., Groothuis, D.G. *et al.* (1985). Water-related nosocomial pneumonia caused by *Legionella pneumophila* serogroup 1 and 10. *J Infect Dis* **152**, 356–63.

Morton, S., Bartlett, C.L.R., Bibby, L.F. *et al.* (1986). An outbreak of Legionnaires' disease from a cooling water system in a power station. *Br J Indust Med* **43**, 630–35.

Muder, R.R., Yu, V.L., McClure, J.K. *et al.* (1983). Nosocomial Legionnaires' disease uncovered in a prospective pneumonia study. *JAMA* **249**, 3184–8.

Neill, M.A., Gorman, G.E., Gilbert, C. *et al.* (1985). Nosocomial legionellosis, Paris, France. *Am J Med* **78**, 581–8.

Nolte, F.S., Conlin, C.A., Roisin, A.J.M. *et al.* (1984). Plasmids as epidemiological markers in nosocomial Legionnaires' disease. *J Infect* **149**, 251–6.

Nordstrom, K., Kallings, I., Dahnsjo, H. *et al.* (1983). An outbreak of Legionnaires' disease in Sweden: Report of sixty-eight cases. *Scand J Infect Dis* **15**, 43–5.

O'Mahony, M., Stanwell-Smith, R., Tillett, H. *et al*. (1986). The Stafford outbreak of Legionnaires' disease. Submitted for publication.

Osterholm, M.T., Chin, T.D.Y., Osborne, D.O. *et al*. (1983). A 1957 outbreak of Legionnaires' disease associated with a meat packing plant. *Am J Epidemiol* **117**, 60–67.

Palmer, S.R., Zamiri, I., Ribeiro, C.D., *et al*. (1986). Legionnaires' disease cluster and reduction in hospital hot water temperatures. *Br Med J* **292**, 1494–5.

Para, M.F., Plouffe, J.F., Maher, W.E. (1984). Production of monoclonal antibodies to *Legionella pneumophila* and relationship of monoclonal binding to plasmid content. In *Legionella. Proceedings of the 2nd International Symposium: Washington, DC.*, pp. 262–4. Edited by Thornsberry, C., Balows, A., Feeley, J.C. and Jakubowski, W.J. Am Soc Microbiol, Washington.

Parry, M.F., Stampleman, L., Hutchinson, J.H. *et al*. (1985). Waterborne *Legionella bozemanii* and nosocomial pneumonia in immunosuppressed patients. *Ann Intern Med* **103**, 205–10.

Plouffe, J., Para, M., Hackman, B. *et al*. (1984). Nosocomial legionnaires' disease: difference in attack rates associated with two strains of *Legionella pneumophila* serogroup 1. In *Legionella. Proceedings of the 2nd International Symposium: Washington, D.C.*, pp. 216–18. Edited by Thornsberry, C., Balows, A., Feeley, J.C. and Jakubowski, W.J. American Society for Microbiology, Washington.

Public Health Laboratory Service. (1985). Communicable Disease Surveillance Centre. CDR 85/50.

Reid, D., Grist, N.R. and Najera, R. (1978). Illness associated with 'package tours': a combined Spanish-Scottish study. *Bull WHO* **56**, 117–22.

Rosmini, F., Castellani-Pastoris, M., Mazzotti, M.F. *et al*. (1984). Febrile illness in successive cohorts of tourists at a hotel on the Italian Adriatic Coast: evidence for a persistent focus of Legionella infection. *Am J Epidemiol* **119**, 124–34.

Rudin, J. and Wing, E.J. (1984). An ongoing outbreak of *Legionella micdadei*. In *Legionella. Proceedings of the 2nd International Symposium: Washington, D.C.*, pp. 227–9. Edited by Thornsberry, C., Balows, A., Feeley, J.C. and Jakubowski, W.J. American Society for Microbiology, Washington.

Schlech III, W.F., Gorman, G.W., Payne, M.C. *et al*. (1985). Legionnaires' disease in the Caribbean. An outbreak associated with a resort hotel. *Arch Intern Med* **145**, 2076–9.

Shands, K.N., Ho, J.L. and Meyer, R.D. (1985). Potable water as a source of Legionnaires' disease. *JAMA* **253**, 1412–16.

Spitalny, K.C., Vogt, R.L., Orciari, L.A. *et al*. (1984). Pontiac fever associated with a whirlpool spa. *Am J Epidemiol* **120**, 809–17.

Stout, J., Yu, V.L. and Vickers, R.M. (1982). Ubiquitousness of *Legionella pneumophila* in the water supply of a hospital with endemic Legionnaires' disease. *New Engl J Med* **306**, 466–8.

Stout, J.E., Yu, V.L. and Best, M.G. (1985). Ecology of *Legionella pneumophila* within water distribution systems. *Appl Environ Microbiol* **49**, 221–8.

Terranova, W., Cohen, M.L. and Fraser, D.W. (1978). 1974 outbreak of Legionnaires' disease diagnosed in 1977. *Lancet* **ii**, 122–4.

Thacker, S.B., Bennett, J.V., Tsai, T.F. *et al*. (1978). An outbreak in 1965 of severe respiratory illness caused by the Legionnaires' disease bacterium. *J Infect Dis* **138**, 512–19.

Timbury, M.C., Donaldson, J.R., McCartney, A.C. *et al*. (1986). Outbreak of legionnaires' disease in Glasgow Royal Infirmary; microbiological aspects. *J. Hyg, Camb*. In press.

Tobin, J.O'H., Bartlett, C.L.R., Waitkins, S.A. *et al*. (1981). Legionnaires' disease: further evidence to implicate water storage and distribution systems as sources. *Br Med J* **282**, 573.

Tobin, J.O'H., Dunhill, M.S., French, M. *et al.* (1980). Legionnaires' disease in a transplant unit: isolation of the causative agent from shower baths. *Lancet* **ii**, 118–21.

Yu, V.L., Zuravleff, J.J., Gavlik, L., *et al.* (1983). Lack of evidence for person-to-person transmission of Legionnaires' disease. *J Infect Dis* **147**, 362.

Zeitler, R., Helms, C., Hall, N. *et al.* (1985). Legionnaires' disease in renal transplant recipients. In *Legionella. Proceedings of the 2nd International Symposium: Washington, DC.*, pp. 234–5. Edited by Thornsberry, C., Balows, A., Feeley, J.C. and Jakubowski, W.J. Am Soc Microbiol, Washington.

Zuravleff, J.J., Yu, V.L., Shonnard, J.W. *et al.* (1983). *Legionella pneumophila* contamination of a hospital humidifier. *Am Rev Respir Dis* **128**, 657–61.

8 Surveillance, Control and Prevention

Surveillance

It is necessary that active surveillance schemes of legionellosis are maintained at local and national level in order to recognize clusters of infections that may have been acquired from common sources. The rapid detection of such clusters should lead to the early identification of the environmental source and the implementation of control measures. Langmuir (1963), has described surveillance as the collection, collation and analysis of data and the prompt dissemination of information to those who need to know so that an action can result. As well as making possible the detection of changes in the pattern of infections this continuous process of surveillance enables the evaluation of specific control and primary preventive measures.

Legionnaires' disease is not a statutory notifiable disease in the UK, although it is in some other countries. There is, however, a scheme for voluntary reporting by microbiology laboratories to the Public Health Laboratory Service Communicable Disease Surveillance Centre in England and Wales; in Scotland infections are reported to the Communicable Diseases (Scotland) Unit (Galbraith, 1982). Medical officers for environmental health in England and Wales are encouraged to report any cases of legionnaires' disease which come to their attention to supplement reporting by the laboratories. In several European and other countries, cases are reported to similar national epidemiological centres or Ministries of Health; in the USA, reporting is to the Centers for Disease Control, Atlanta.

In England and Wales, surveillance of legionella infections is operated through a national laboratory reporting scheme. About 400 microbiological laboratories voluntarily report the identification of legionella and other infections weekly to the PHLS Communicable Disease Surveillance Centre. Locally recognized clusters or unusual incidents may be reported at any time by telephone or telex. On receipt of the report a questionnaire is sent by CDSC to the microbiologist or physician in charge of the case to obtain additional information. If a clinical specimen has been sent to a PHLS reference laboratory to confirm the diagnosis, then this laboratory sends out the questionnaire. Details are sought on recent hospital admissions, travel and employment to enable the recognition of nosocomial clusters and clusters associated with hotels and places of work. Whenever possible, any identified clusters are investigated by the Public Health Laboratory Service

Table 8.1 Clusters of cases of legionnaires' disease associated with buildings in England and Wales 1979–1982. From Bartlett, C.L.R. and Bibby, L.F., 1983

Establishments	Number of clusters*	Number of cases	Clusters with cases in more than one year
Hotels	24	107	17
Hospitals	7	26	2
Other	1	3	–
Total	32	136	19

* Two or more cases

in collaboration with local hospital microbiologists and public health authorities. Bartlett and Bibby (1983), reviewed the data collected in this manner for cases reported in England and Wales during the 4-year period 1979–1982. The majority of the 588 cases of legionella pneumonia reported during this period appeared to be sporadic, but 32 clusters of two or more cases were identified through national surveillance (Table 8.1). Most clusters were associated with hotels, all but two of which were in tourist resorts abroad. Seven clusters were associated with hospitals and one with an industrial site. The surveillance scheme demonstrated that some buildings would provide a source of infection over several years unless control measures were implemented. Remarkably 17 of the 24 hotels implicated as sources of infection were associated with cases in more than one year. One hotel is known to have been responsible for cases of legionnaires' disease over 7 years (Bartlett *et al.*, 1984). From 1977–1985, 48 clusters of legionnaires' disease were recognized (PHLS unpublished information) and the epidemiological investigation of several of these led to the identification of environmental sources and the development of effective control measures.

Active surveillance at local level is important to determine the pattern of endemic legionella infections and to recognize the occurrence of clusters in time and place. Outbreaks in hospitals are usually first recognized locally but outbreaks associated with hotels are detected mainly through national surveillance. Geographical clusters in the community may be readily recognized at an early stage if records are kept of postcodes of home and work addresses. Indeed, a common postal code on the laboratory form was the essential clue that lead to the detection of a recent outbreak in Glasgow (Ad-Hoc Committee, 1986).

In the absence of precise epidemiological markers, such as might be provided by a well validated subtyping scheme for *L. pneumophila*, it is not possible to identify unequivocally the source of a sporadic infection. It is well worthwhile, however, keeping a list of buildings possibly associated with legionella infections because some establishments may continue to serve as sources intermittently over a long period of time. By careful review of surveillance data it may be possible to recognize such sources even in the absence of clustering in time.

Epidemiological investigations which are indicated when an apparently sporadic case of legionnaires' disease is recognized

The first steps in the investigation are to confirm the diagnosis and to take a detailed history from the person with legionnaires' disease, or from a relative. A history of any travel away from home during the 10 days before onset should be sought, and the travel itineraries recorded. Any hospital visits during the same period or attendances at conferences or other functions should also be noted, as should recreational activities, occupation and place of work.

If the person was in hospital throughout the 10 days prior to onset of legionella pneumonia, then it is probable that the infection was nosocomial ie. hospital acquired. A search should be made for other cases by reviewing all pneumonias acquired in the hospital in the recent past; legionella serology should be done if an aetiology has not been established. Stored serum samples, perhaps taken for virology or antibiotic assay, may be available from earlier cases. The hospital microbiologists and clinicians should be informed so that they can look out for new cases. Sputum or samples of lower respiratory tract secretions should be cultured for legionella in any newly presenting nosocomial pneumonias in the hospital. The question of environmental sampling will be discussed in the next section.

In cases of community acquired pneumonia, the history may give a clue as to the source. If the person had stayed in a hotel or similar establishment then the local and national surveillance data should be checked to see if other cases have been reported in association with the building. Any general practitioners serving the hotel should also be consulted. It would also be worth questioning the hotel's management to see if they are aware of other pneumonia cases among residents or staff.

If no other related cases are found, no further steps need be taken other than to ensure that the hotel's or hospital's engineer is following good engineering practices in the maintenance and operation of the various building services including water systems. These practices are covered in national guidelines issued to hospital engineers by the Department of Health and Social Security in England and Wales, the Welsh Office and the Scottish Home and Health Office; the last section of this chapter discusses such preventive measures.

Work colleagues of the person who has developed legionnaires' disease may present problems for public health authorities. Often in the past the assumption has been made by fellow employees that the work place was the likely source of infection, although in practice this has rarely been shown to be so. Unrealistic demands have been made on occasion for eradication of legionellas from the site. Fortunately, such demands have been fairly easily overcome by means of careful explanation of the known sources of legionella and modes of transmission. Enquiries should be made of the occupational physician or medical advisor, to determine whether there have been other pneumonias among the work force. If there is no medical advisor to the establishment then the personnel officer will usually have records of sickness absence. Again, it is important to ensure that the maintenance of any water systems capable of producing aerosols is in keeping with the national guide-lines for the prevention of legionnaires' disease.

Commercial whirlpools or spas have been shown to serve as sources of legionnaires' disease, so if the person who developed legionnaires' disease is known to have used such a pool, similar enquiries should be made to look for related cases. In the absence of other cases the public health authority should make sure that the maintenance of the pool is satisfactory and that a log is kept of the chemical treatment and any test results.

Environmental investigations which are indicated when a sporadic case of legionnaires' disease is recognized

In general, if a sporadic case of legionnaires' disease is reported and enquiries fail to find related cases, then sampling for microbiology in the home, work place or other buildings visited by the person, is not indicated. This is because surveys have shown that *L. pneumophila* can be expected to be found in the water systems of most buildings. Finding the organism would not, therefore, demonstrate the source of infection and furthermore, negative results could give a false sense of security.

There are, however, two possible exceptions to this rule at present and the advice could be further modified with advances in microbiological methods. Firstly, some would argue that any one case developing in a patient who had been in hospital for more than 10 days warrants extensive sampling of all potential environmental sources of legionella, followed by the application of control measures. The problem with such an approach is that the micro-biological investigations are unlikely to reliably identify the source and the maintenance of long term control measures to all sites found to be positive may be costly and unnecessary. If the infecting organism is an unusual sero-group of *L. pneumophila* or another species of legionella then it may be pos-sible to identify the likely source of infection. This is especially so if the diag-nosis has been made by culturing the organism from the patient, rather than by serology or other method, because the clinical and environmental isolates can be compared in the laboratory. This will be useful for those serotypes of *L. pneumophila* and other legionella species which are only rarely found in environmental samples. Even for *L. pneumophila* serogroup 1, the com-monest cause of legionnaires' disease, with the development of well validated subtyping schemes using monoclonal antibodies or isoenzymes, or perhaps with the use of specific genetic probes or the recognition of virulence markers, it may be possible to identify the probable source with more confi-dence, even for sporadic cases. In the long term, the development of such techniques may even permit the localization of sources of sporadic infection in the home or work place.

Epidemiological investigations which are indicated when a cluster of cases of legionnaires' disease is recognized

The same basic principles should be followed in the epidemiological inves-tigation of legionellosis as for any other cluster or outbreak of communicable disease. The first key steps in the process include confirmation of diagnosis, the establishment of a case definition for epidemiological purposes, the confirmation of the existence of an outbreak, a search for other related cases followed by a description of the characteristics of all those who are affected and their distribution in time and place.

This first part of the investigation is known as the descriptive epidemiology which, when completed, often provides clues as to the possible sources and modes of transmission. The second stage, or analytical epidemiology, sets out to test the hypotheses that are put forward during the initial investigation. The approach generally is to make a comparison between the people who were affected and a sample of those that remained well. This will often lead to the identification of sources which may be confirmed by microbiology. Tracer studies may be used to verify the mode of transmission.

The steps in the investigation of an outbreak will now be considered in more detail.

Confirmation of diagnosis
The diagnosis should be verified as soon as possible, ideally by culture of the organism. Legionellas may be isolated from sputum, or occasionally blood, although the recovery rate is greater from secretions taken from the lower respiratory tract at endoscopy or by bronchial lavage or tracheal aspiration. Alternatively, the diagnosis may be confirmed by the demonstration of a four-fold or greater rise in specific antibody titre. A rapid microagglutination test and an immunofluorescent antibody test (IFAT) are readily available for this purpose in Britain. If an acute serum specimen has not been collected then a convalescent IFAT titre of 128 or greater is generally accepted as being indicative of recent legionella infection if the clinical features are compatible with legionnaires' disease. Less than 1 per cent of the population in England and Wales have IFAT titres of 64 or more against the formolised yolk sac antigen issued by the Division of Microbiological Reagents and Quality Control, Central Public Health Laboratory, Colindale, London NW9.

Case definition
Because attempts to isolate *L. pneumophila* from sputum have tended to be unsuccessful and many physicians are reluctant to use invasive methods to obtain specimens from the lower respiratory tract, the diagnosis of legionnaires' disease is often established on the basis of serology. Several weeks may elapse between onset of illness and seroconversion. This delay creates a problem for the epidemiologist during the early stages of an outbreak investigation and may necessitate the use of an initial definition based solely on clinical findings.

Such a definition usually hinges on the clinical and radiological findings which are indicative of pneumonia. This approach had to be used during the original outbreak among American Legion delegates in Philadelphia in 1976, when the aetiology was not known (Fraser *et al.*, 1977). The clinical criteria selected then required that a person have onset, during the 18 day epidemic period, of an illness characterized by cough and fever (temperature of 38.9°C or higher) or any fever and chest x-ray evidence of pneumonia. Using this definition the investigators were able to demonstrate that legionnaires' disease was not spread from person-to-person but was probably acquired from a common environmental source by means of airborne transmission.

It is always important to include a clinical component in the case definition, particularly if the diagnosis is made by serology because no such test is likely to be fully sensitive. In the epidemiological investigation of an outbreak of legionnaires' disease among tourists who had stayed at a hotel in Spain, clinical or radiological evidence of pneumonia was accepted as the case definition (Bartlett *et al.*, 1984). Fifty-nine cases of pneumonia were identified but in only 25 of these was there supporting laboratory evidence of legionella infection. The distribution of cases over time in those individuals who could give an exact date of onset is shown in Figure 8.1. This 'epidemic curve' shows a temporal clustering of legionnaires' disease and other pneumonia cases. Only one or two cases of pneumonia at most would have been expected in the population at risk during the period of the outbreak. This suggests that nearly all, if not all, the pneumonia cases in guests were part of the same epidemic and probably acquired from the same source. There are several possible explanations of the fact that not all were positive for legionella infection. Perhaps all the pneumonias were due to *L. pneumophila* serogroup 1, but the serological tests had failed to identify them or, more likely, some of the infections may have been due to other serogroups or other species of legionella not recognized with the existing serological tests. One further possibility which should be borne in mind is that the pneumonias may have been caused by organisms other than members of the family Legionellaceae but acquired from the same environmental source. It is not possible to answer this question at present but specimens have been stored and will be re-examined as new agents are reported.

In small outbreaks the inclusion of clinical as well as laboratory confirmed cases may help initially by increasing the number of subjects in the investigation and thus improve the statistical power in analytical studies, thereby facilitating the demonstration of an association with an environmental source. In these circumstances the analysis should be repeated when case-searching is completed, and if there are sufficient cases, using only those having both clinical and laboratory evidence of infection.

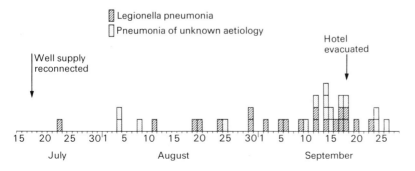

Fig. 8.1 Outbreak of legionnaires' disease associated with a hotel in Spain. Epidemic curve for 37 cases of pneumonia, July to September 1980. From Bartlett *et al.*,1984.

Confirmation of the existence of an outbreak

There are several definitions of an outbreak, but perhaps the most useful is the one which states that an outbreak is present when the observed rate of a disease exceeds the expected rate. This definition draws attention to the importance of maintaining surveillance to collect baseline data on the frequency of disease. Such data may not be readily available for legionnaires' disease and any local surveillance data may underestimate the incidence of legionnaires' disease. Not uncommonly, the infection may be overlooked by clinicians when considering the differential diagnosis of pneumonia and appropriate specimens may not be collected to enable the establishment of the laboratory diagnosis. When a case is recognized this may lead to a greater awareness of the infection locally and consequently to greater detection of the endemic level of infection. A recent multi-centre study of pneumonia in Britain found that only about 2 per cent of primary community acquired pneumonias requiring admission to hospital were due to *L. pneumophila* (British Thoracic Society and Public Health Laboratory Service, 1986). A distinct clustering of two or more cases in time and place in any one locality is therefore suggestive of a common source outbreak.

Case searching

Because clinical recognition of legionnaires' disease is often poor, active case searching is usually necessary to determine the extent of an outbreak. The recognition of early cases, which may have been overlooked at the time may provide clues as to the source of infection. Furthermore, the task of demonstrating an epidemiological association with a suspected source may be made easier if a larger number of cases is available for study. For example, in an investigation of an outbreak of legionnaires' disease among persons who had stayed in a hotel, 21 of 26 cases of pneumonia, 16 of whom had serological evidence of legionella infection, were identified as a result of retrospective case-searching (Communicable Disease Surveillance Centre, 1985). With this number of infections, it was possible to demonstrate in a case control study a highly significant association with use of the whirlpool spas in the hotel and together with the microbiological evidence demonstrate convincingly that these pools were the source of the outbreak. The methods used for case-searching included a review of current and earlier admissions to the local hospital and the follow up of a cohort of guests who had stayed at the hotel since it had opened for the season. At a national level, the outbreak was reported on the front page of the Communicable Disease Report with a request for information on any other cases of pneumonia among recent visitors to Brighton; several cases, all of whom had stayed at the one hotel, were identified by this means.

The CDR is a weekly report which is sent to infectious disease physicians, microbiologists, community physicians, environmental health officers and others, many of whom have responded in the past to requests for reports on a variety of possible associated infections. In the investigation of the outbreak associated with the hotel in Benidorm, Spain in 1980, a similar request for information in the CDR led to the recognition of 64 cases of pneumonia among recent visitors to the resort (Bartlett *et al.*, 1984). Fifty-nine of these pneumonias were in guests who had stayed at one hotel, thus providing a clue as to the likely source of the infection.

In the hospital setting, a retrospective search for cases may be readily undertaken if the infection control team have maintained active clinical surveillance of nosocomial lower respiratory tract infections. In Britain, surveillance of nosocomial infection is largely based on laboratory reports and only a small number of hospitals will have clinical surveillance data. Under these circumstances, a retrospective search may be made of case notes or duplicate copies of x-ray reports held in the radiology department but these activities can be extremely time consuming. With limited reserves, efforts can be concentrated on the records of those patients who were likely to have been at greatest risk of developing legionnaires' disease. Palmer and colleagues (1986), adopted this approach in the investigation of a cluster of cases in a hospital in Wales. They studied patients who had received steroids or cytotoxic drugs or suffered from diabetes. The detection by these means of a distinct cluster of cases in time led to the identification of the hot water system as the source of infection.

Another method proved particularly useful in the investigation of legionnaires' disease in Kingston-upon-Thames hospital in 1980 (Fisher-Hoch *et al.*, 1981). The question that needed to be answered was whether the hospital's hot water system or its cooling water system was the source of the outbreak. On this occasion, cases of legionnaires' disease were sought retrospectively by examining stored specimens of lung taken at post-mortem and serum specimens which had been collected for virology or antibiotic assay. The latter approach proved successful in identifying three patients who had acquired their infection in hospital during the winter months before the cooling tower had been brought into operation.

Descriptive epidemiology
Detailed case histories should be taken from all those persons fulfilling the case definition or from their relatives or friends. From these histories one should attempt to determine the personal characteristics of cases; in other words, ask the question, who was affected? It is customary to present the age and sex distribution of cases because these are two of the most important factors influencing the occurrence of disease. The time of life at which an infectious disease predominates is influenced by such factors as the degree of exposure to the agent at various ages, variations in susceptibility with age and the duration of the immunity developed after infection (Friedman, 1974). In the investigation of the outbreak associated with the American Legion Convention in Philadelphia in 1976, it was found that the attack rate increased dramatically with age (Fraser *et al.*, 1977). The ages of the delegates were analysed in 10-year age bands and it was found that the proportion of those affected increased successively with each age band after the age of 40. Many other investigations have found that the middle-aged and elderly are most at risk of acquiring legionnaires' disease.

It is worth dwelling for a moment on the concept of considering the entire population at risk (be it cohort of hotel guests, hospital patients or conference attenders) and the calculation of attack rates. Reference has already been made to age and sex specific attack rates but the calculation may be made on any other relevant variable, such as time or place. Rates are calculated because a study of the numerator data alone may be misleading. An obvious example would be the comparison of the distribution of cases in two geographical areas. An excess of cases in one area might merely reflect the fact that more people live there. A higher attack rate in that locality, however, might warrant further investigation.

Other personal characteristics which are used when describing the distribution of disease are occupation, ethnic group and social class, but there is little in the literature to indicate their importance as determinants of legionellosis. Although no particular occupational group has been identified as being at a significantly greater risk of acquiring legionellosis than any other, detailed work histories should be taken. Water is used in various processes in many industries and some of these so called 'process waters' may represent potential sources of legionella infection. So far, only cooling water systems and water based lubricants have been implicated in an industrial setting, but the possibility that other process waters might be responsible should not be overlooked.

The determination of the distribution of cases in place and time are the next steps to be taken in the descriptive epidemiology. Observations on where and when people were affected often serve as a pointer to the source of the outbreak. Histories should be taken of the places visited during the time range of the incubation period, which in legionnaires' disease is 2-10 days and in Pontiac fever 4-66 hours. Specific enquiries should be made about visiting or staying in hotels, hospitals, conference centres or recreational facilities likely to have whirlpools or spas. In an investigation of an outbreak of legionnaires' disease in the USA in 1978, 47 cases were found at three hospitals in two states (Dondero *et al.*, 1980). Remarkably, 39 patients (85 per cent) had an association with one hospital in the city of Memphis during the 10 days before onset of their illness, either as patients, employees, visitors or passers by. A cooling tower in the grounds of the hospital was eventually shown to be the source of infection. A study of those persons who acquired legionnaires' disease as inpatients, found clustering in one wing of the hospital. Attack rates were calculated and the highest rates were found in rooms which were ventilated with air which was drawn from near the cooling tower (see Fig. 7.6). The distribution of cases, particularly when expressed as a rate, was particularly helpful in this instance in identifying the mode of transmission. There are several other examples in which a study of the distribution of cases in relation to building services pointed to the source of infection.

In an outbreak of nosocomial legionnaires' disease in a hospital in France, three patients developed legionellosis within the same 24 hour period (Neill *et al.*, 1985). All had been in the same wing, although on different floors, but it was found that their rooms were supplied with hot water by one of 18 hot water pipes that serve the patient floors. The probability of this association with a single pipe occurring by chance was estimated at 3 in a 1000, suggesting that this observation was highly significant. The hot water system was later shown convincingly to be the source.

Negative information may also be useful. The investigators of an outbreak of legionnaires' disease associated with a hotel in Spain had to consider the possibility of a nearby cooling tower being the source (Bartlett *et al.*, 1984). They found the attack rates were no greater among guests who had stayed in

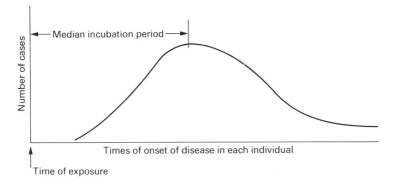

Fig. 8.2 Distribution of times of onset of disease (the epidemic curve) and median incubation period in a point source outbreak.
Adapted from Lilienfeld, 1976.

bedrooms facing the cooling tower or those in the two wings next to it. This tended to exclude the cooling tower as the source and indeed, the hotel's domestic water system was shown to be responsible for the outbreak.

Plotting the time distribution is often as informative as and complementary to determining the distribution by place. It is customary to present the data as a histogram with number of cases on the y-axis and time on the x-axis (Fig. 8.2). The distribution of cases on the graph is commonly referred to as the epidemic curve. A point source outbreak is characterized by a sharp rise in the number of cases over time followed often by a somewhat longer fall. Such an epidemic curve was found with cases among American Legion conventioneers (Fig. 8.3) during the investigation of the outbreak in Philadelphia in 1976 (Fraser *et al.*, 1977). More commonly the epidemic curve for

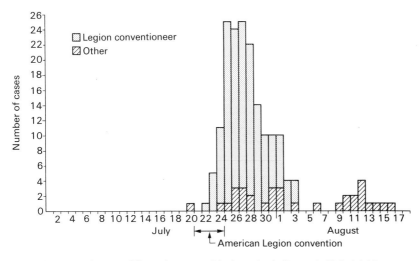

Fig. 8.3 Dates of onset of illness in cases of legionnaires' disease in Philadelphia, July 1 – August 18, 1976. Dates of onset of two cases of legionnaires' disease are unknown. From Fraser *et al.*, 1977.

legionnaires' disease extends over a longer time period and reflects a continuing common source of infection. An extreme example of this pattern (see Fig. 7.2) is given in the account of an outbreak of legionnaires' disease in the Wadsworth Memorial Hospital in Los Angeles (Shands *et al.*, 1985).

In a true point source outbreak the epidemic curve reflects the distribution of incubation periods. The median point on the curve represents the median incubation period (Fig. 8.2). It is therefore possible to estimate the time when the infections were contracted and enquiries about environmental exposures at that time may provide pointers to the source. Whatever the shape of the epidemic curve it is often helpful to mark on the figure, events or exposures which may be related to the occurrence of disease. For example, in the Wadsworth Memorial Hospital a distinct wave of cases followed a sudden fall in the pressure in the hospital's domestic water system (see Fig. 7.2). The hospital's water system was eventually shown to be the source of the outbreak (Shands *et al.*, 1985). On the epidemic curve of the Memphis Hospital outbreak (see Fig. 7.5), the period of operation of an auxilliary cooling tower is shown. The first cases occurred shortly after the tower was brought into use and the last case occurred 9 days after it was shut down, which is within the upper limit of the incubation period. The close temporal relationship between the operation of this equipment and the distribution of cases strongly suggests its involvement in the incident.

In other outbreaks the link with the environmental factor has been less striking, but has still provided a valuable clue to the source. In the Benidorm hotel outbreak, the first case occurred shortly after a supplementary well water supply was reconnected (Fig. 8.1). It is open to speculation whether this reconnection seeded the hotel's domestic water system with legionella or merely provided chemical or other nutritional factors which enabled the organism to proliferate. Either way a plausible explanation is provided as to the onset of the outbreak.

When completed, the descriptive epidemiology in conjunction with the results of microbiological examination of environmental samples will often point clearly to the source of infection and mode of transmission. It must be borne in mind, however, that any such conclusion is based only on circumstantial evidence which may be misleading. Control measures have often been applied on the basis of such observations and in most cases these have been successful. On occasions though, the wrong conclusion was drawn and ineffective but costly control measures applied. Whenever practicable, the circumstantial evidence produced at this stage should be tested by means of an analytical epidemiological study and microbiological studies of the environment.

Analytical epidemiology

On the basis of the descriptive epidemiology, hypotheses should be formulated on the source of infection and mode of transmission. These may be tested by means of either a case control study or (historical) cohort study. A third approach, the intervention study is really excluded on ethical grounds in the investigation of legionnaires' disease. Only an outline will be given of each type of study and readers should refer to a textbook on epidemiology for a comprehensive description of the methods.

In a case control or retrospective study, people with the disease (cases) are compared with persons who do not have the disease (controls). The object is to compare the numbers in each group that are exposed or not exposed to the putative source. For example, in the investigation of the outbreak of legionnaires' disease among persons who had stayed at a hotel in Brighton (Public Health Laboratory Service, 1985) the descriptive epidemiology suggested that the infection may have been linked with bathing in either of the hotel's whirlpools. The so-called 'null hypothesis' was that there was no difference in the proportion of cases or controls who had used either whirlpool. The results of the microbiological studies had not identified a single potential source because *L. pneumophila* serogroup 1, the causative agent, had been isolated from the hotel's hot water system, cold water system and both whirlpools. The results of the case control study are shown in Table 8.2. A highly significant association was found with the use of either whirlpool and with use of individual whirlpools. The final column shows the probability of such a result occurring by chance. Various statistical tests may be applied to determine probability in the case control study; in this case the Fisher's exact test was used. The Chi-squared test is commonly used but if cases and controls have been matched for one or more variable, such as age, then other types of tests are more appropriate.

In the Brighton study an association was also found with using the swimming pool, but it was considered that this was because whirlpool users also tended to bathe in the swimming pool. An attempt was made to demonstrate an independent effect of bathing in whirlpools but the numbers were too small to permit this. Unlike the whirlpools, the swimming pool had been well maintained and a log kept of daily test results for free residual chlorine levels. These had always been satisfactory as had routine microbiological tests for water quality. *L. pneumophila* was not isolated from the swimming pool and it was concluded that the whirlpools which did yield the organism were the source of the outbreak.

In a (historical) cohort study, a population is studied over a period of time. All should be free of the disease at the beginning of the study period but individuals may vary in their exposure to the suspected source. With this method, the group exposed to the source and the group not exposed are studied to

Table 8.2 History of exposure to potential sources of legionella in 21 cases of pneumonia and unmatched controls. From Public Health Laboratory Service, 1985

| | Cases | | Controls | | Fishers exact |
	Exposed	Not exposed	Exposed	Not exposed	*probability
Wall whirlpool	13	8	18	52	0.006
Centre whirlpool	12	9	12	55	0.002
Either whirlpool +	17	4	20	47	0.00008
Swimming pool	15	6	19	45	0.002
Bath	11	9	37	15	NS
Shower	2	17	14	39	NS
Drinking tap water	8	12	37	35	NS

* 2-tailed
+ odds ratio for either whirlpool use (estimate of relative risk) = 10 (95 % confidence limits 3–35)

determine the proportion in each who develop the disease. When investigating legionnaires' disease, the epidemiologist can study all those staying at a hotel or in a hospital during the epidemic period. In cohort studies, larger numbers of persons have to be studied and an ascertainment made of the presence of infection in each. It may be difficult to locate all subjects and this type of study tends to be costly and time consuming. Its major advantages are the ability to calculate incidence rates and relative risk. The relative risk is calculated by dividing the incidence rate among those exposed by the incidence rate among the unexposed.

In case control studies it is possible to calculate the odds ratio, which is an estimate of relative risk, but because the number of subjects studied is often small the confidence interval may be large. For example, in the Brighton study the odds-ratio for either whirlpool use was calculated as 10 but the 95 per cent confidence limits were 3–35.

Environmental investigations which are indicated when a cluster of cases of legionnaires' disease is recognized

It is often possible at an early stage of the epidemiological investigation to locate a building which contains the probable reservoir of infection, although the precise source may not be identified until much later. Commonly the building is a hotel or hospital, but it might be a factory or some other type of establishment. At the outset, water samples for microbiological examination should be collected from all known potential sources of legionella, such as hot and cold water and any cooling water systems. Any water systems capable of producing airborne water droplets should be considered as potential sources. The optimum volume of water to be collected from each site is unclear but in Britain it has been conventional practice to take 5 litre samples. This water is then subjected to membrane filtration in the laboratory.

Hot water systems appear to be the most important sources of outbreaks of legionnaires' disease, at least in Europe. Samples should be taken from the mains supply, any holding tanks, the calorifier (heating cylinder) drain, and from hot taps and showers. If there is a recirculating hot water system then samples should be taken from the nearest outlet to the calorifier and another outlet at the return end of the loop. This is done because there may be a fall in the water temperature as it circulates around the building and the growth of legionella is dependent on temperature. The water temperature should be taken from each site examined, once the sample has been collected.

At hot water taps, the temperature should be recorded immediately after sampling and then 3 minutes after flushing to obtain a reading which is more representative of the circulating hot water. A large temperature gradient may be found if the tap is on the end of a long spur (deadleg) of pipework. The pH and free residual chlorine level should also be recorded. Cold water samples should be collected from the rising main, any holding tank and from taps and showers. It is important that samples should be taken from hot and cold taps and any shower units used by patients prior to their onset of legionnaires' disease. This is necessary because there may be localized growth of legionella in the peripheral part of the water system.

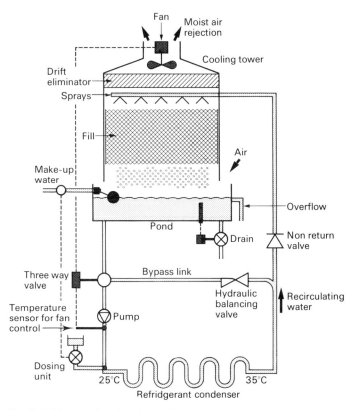

Fig. 8.4 Diagram showing the cooling water system pipework found in a cooling tower.

If a cooling tower or evaporative condenser is a potential source then samples should be taken from the pond, the cooling water return at the top of the tower, and, if possible, points in the pipe-work which carries the circulating cooling water (Fig. 8.4). Samples from the cooling water system pipework are particularly important if there is a bypass loop, because temperatures which favour the rapid multiplication of legionella may be sustained in this part of the system. If whirlpools or humidifiers are thought to be possible sources then their water supply should be sampled as should any reservoirs or filters.

A clear relationship between total microbial counts and the presence of legionellas has not been demonstrated, but it may be helpful to take samples for routine microbiology (HMSO) as well as for legionella culture. This is certainly necessary if the inspection of the building services suggests that good engineering practices have not been followed in maintaining the water systems. In the outbreak of legionnaires' disease from the whirlpool spas in Brighton, high counts of *E. coli* were obtained and *Pseudomonas aeruginosa* was isolated. This substantiated other observations that the pools had not been correctly treated and maintained, and could have been the source of the outbreak. Once the exact source of an outbreak has been located through epidemiological studies further sampling for legionella culture should take place at intervals to ensure that the control measures which have been applied are effective in controlling the growth of the organism.

Once control measures have been established it has been the practice in Britain to sample at monthly intervals for 6 months and thereafter less frequently. The efficacy of the control measures should also be monitored by means of continuing active surveillance for legionnaires' disease.

Control measures

This section deals with the treatment of water systems which have been shown to be the source of a cluster or outbreak of legionnaires' disease by means of epidemiological and microbiological studies. The control measures which have been developed in recent years were applied largely on an empirical basis in the late 1970s and early 1980s when environmental sources were only beginning to be recognized. The various methods used for control have been refined over the years but as yet there is no good data to show which method is the most effective over a long period of time.

Domestic hot water systems in large buildings

Domestic hot water systems in large buildings appear, at least in Britain, to be the most important source of endemic and epidemic legionella infections. This source was first recognized in the investigation of two nosocomial cases of legionnaires' disease in Oxford (Tobin *et al.*, 1980). Shock chlorination (super chlorination) was the control method which was used on that occasion. The cold water supply tank was drained, then filled with water containing 50 mg/litre (ppm) of free residual chlorine and left to stand for 3 hours. The tank was then drained again, cleaned and refilled with similarly chlorinated water which was run into the cold water system where it was held for a further 3 hours before being flushed out. The hot water system was treated in a similar fashion and the use of shower units was prohibited. These methods appeared to be effective in preventing further cases but 9 months later *L. pneumophila* was again isolated from the water system.

To control an outbreak the same year from a hotel's domestic water system, continuous treatment methods were used (Tobin *et al.*, 1981). Shock chlorination and cleaning of the hot and cold water systems similar to the methods used in Oxford was undertaken and then a sodium hypochlorite solution injection unit was installed to achieve continuous chlorination. The object was to obtain levels of 1–2 mg/litre (ppm) at all outlets. After initial adjustments it became possible to maintain free chlorine levels within this range at cold water taps but not at hot water taps without producing unacceptably high levels in the cold water system. To overcome this problem the hot water temperature was raised to give, in effect, an intermittent pasteurization effect. It was recommended that the circulating hot water temperature should be maintained within the range 50–60°C; the upper limit was set because of the risk of scalding. There is a smaller risk of scalding from water at temperatures between 50 and 60°C, but no incidents have occurred in several hospitals and hotels which have followed this control measure for more than 5 years.

The following year, a middle aged man developed legionnaires' disease 5 days after staying at the hotel and it was discovered that he had occupied one of the three rooms in which it had not been possible to achieve a minimum temperature of 50°C (Bartlett and Bibby, 1983). *L. pneumophila* was isolated from water samples taken from the hot water tap in the man's room but not from other parts of the hot water system. It was concluded that raising the temperature of the circulating hot water system alone in buildings might not be successful in controlling legionella, particularly if there are 'deadlegs' arising from the loop. To overcome this problem a second sodium hypochlorite solution injection unit was fitted to the hot water pipe-work in the 'flow' part of the circuit. This part of the pipe-work carries water which has just been heated in the calorifier.

With the installation of this second unit it has been possible to maintain levels of free residual chlorine of 1–2 mg/litre (ppm) at hot water taps as well. No cases have been detected in association with the hotel since then.

Similar methods were used to control an outbreak of legionnaires' disease in Kingston-upon-Thames Hospital (Fisher-Hoch *et al.*, 1981). These measures were successful until a year later when another case occurred in the hospital. It was concluded that he had contracted the infection on the day in which a reserve calorifier had been brought into use (Fisher-Hoch *et al.*, 1982). This calorifier had had its heating coil switched off, but remained filled with water so that it was immediately available for use whenever needed. The stagnant water in the calorifier was implicated as the source through microbiological studies and metal content analyses of samples taken from the calorifier and the taps and shower used by the patient. This incident and the findings of a survey of hotels, hospitals, office blocks and other large buildings (Bartlett *et al.*, 1986) indicate that calorifiers may be important reservoirs of legionella. Consequently control measures in the long term should include at least once yearly draining down and cleaning of the calorifiers. Furthermore, if calorifiers have been held on standby, they should be drained down and flushed with chlorinated water prior to being brought back into use. Ideally, the calorifier containing the fresh chlorinated water should be held overnight before use to allow the settling of any suspended sediment which may have arisen through the flushing. This procedure would also be advisable following routine cleaning of the calorifier.

Elsewhere, continuous chlorination alone has been used to control outbreaks of nosocomial legionnaires' disease but generally this has been less effective than a combination of continuous chlorination and raising of hot water temperatures.

In the Wadsworth Memorial Hospital, a minimum level of 2 mg/litre (ppm) of free residual chlorine was maintained in the hospital's water from late July 1980 (Shands *et al.*, 1985). Nevertheless, it can be seen from the epidemic curve (see Fig. 7.2, p. 97), that further cases occurred in late 1980 and during 1981.

Baird and colleagues (1984), chlorinated continuously the water supply to a hospital in Columbus, Ohio, USA to control a high level of endemic legionellosis. A level of 4 mg/litre of free residual chlorine was maintained over a 1 year study period but *L. pneumophila* was not eradicated from the hot water tanks or other parts of the water system. A reduction was seen, however, in the frequency of isolation of *L. pneumophila* from taps and showers. Furthermore, there was a significant decrease in the incidence of nosocomial legionellosis, although seven cases were recognized during the study period. It is unclear whether these infections were acquired from the domestic hot water system, but if so, raising the hot water temperatures as well may have improved the effectiveness of the control measures.

Massanari and colleagues (1984), used higher levels of chlorination to control an outbreak (Helms *et al.*, 1983) in a large University hospital in Iowa, USA. Following initial shock chlorination and raising the temperature in the hospital's hot water system from 41–64°C for 41 days, they installed continuous flow-adjusted chlorinators to both the hot and cold water systems. Over a period of 16 months they maintained chlorine levels at 8 mg/litre (range 2.5–15 mg/litre) in the hot water and 7.3 mg/litre (range 2.0–15 mg/litre) in the cold water. During this time only two of 355 water samples grew *L. pneumophila* and these two samples were collected from rooms which had been vacant for at least a month. It was presumed that the residual chlorine had dissipated in the stagnant water and a policy was introduced in the hospital of flushing water outlets in rooms vacant for more than 48 hours. No new cases of nosocomial legionnaires' disease occurred during the 16 months. No engineering problems were reported and the unusually high levels of chlorine were said to be acceptable to patients and staff.

Experience has shown, therefore, that continuous chlorination is a relatively inexpensive and effective measure although some failures can be expected unless high levels of free residual chlorine are maintained at all outlets. The main disadvantage of continuous chlorination in the long term is the acceleration of metal corrosion which will take place, particularly in hot water circuits. This could present problems in just a few years if chlorination is maintained at the levels used in Iowa, especially if the water naturally has corrosive characteristics due to its chemical composition. On the other hand, there are several buildings in England in which free residual chlorine levels of between 1 and 2 mg/litre (ppm) have been maintained for more than 5 years without the development of significant corrosion. Another concern is the possibility that continuous chlorination in a hospital will raise the level of chlorinated organic compounds such as trihalomethanes in the water, but the extent and any effect remain to be evaluated. It should be stressed at this point that it is important to maintain the pH of water within the range 7.2–7.8; this will not only ensure the availability of free chlorine but also minimize the production of trihalomethanes and possibly provide a less than optimal pH for the multiplication of legionella.

One other method for controlling the growth of the organism in hot water systems which has been used successfully, consists of flushing intermittently the entire system with water heated to temperatures up to 77°C. Best and colleagues (1983), were the first to use this approach to control an outbreak of nosocomial legionellosis due to *L. pneumophila* and *L. micdadei*. They developed a system of raising the temperature in the hot water storage tanks from 70–77°C and holding at this level for 3 days. The hot water temperature was then allowed to return to the original 45°C but the procedure was repeated at intervals depending on the results of surveillance cultures. During the intermittent boosting of the hot water tank temperatures, all taps and showers in the patient areas were flushed on two occasions, 24 hours apart, for 30 minutes. Exposure to this very hot water could cause scalding in a matter of seconds but Best and colleagues reported that no incidents had occurred during the first 18 months evaluation of their control method. Patients and staff were alerted to the risk by means of the hospital daily bulletin and signs at every water outlet. The control measures did not eliminate the organisms from the water system, although the frequency with which they were isolated from water samples was reduced. In association with this reduction was a fall in the number of legionella infections but nosocomial legionellosis was not entirely prevented.

Rudin and Wing (1984), also used intermittent raising of hot water temperatures to control an outbreak of legionellosis caused by *L. micdadei*. They chose lower temperatures, raising the hot water temperature from 43°C to only 54°C. This was done on a bimonthly basis and at the same time the entire system was flushed for approximately 30 minutes. Sediment from the hot water tanks was drained weekly. Despite these measures, cases of *L. micdadei* pneumonia continued to occur, often with distinct clustering in time. No other reservoirs of *L. micdadei* were found in the hospital, so it seems reasonable to conclude that intermittent flushing with water at 54°C is not an effective control measure.

Meenhorst and colleagues (1985), adopted yet another approach to control a nosocomial outbreak of legionellosis due to *L. pneumophila* serogroups 1 and 10. Their strategy consisted of raising the hot water temperature permanently in combination with regular flushing of taps and showers. Water in the hot tanks was held at 72°C and this achieved temperatures at most outlets of at least 60°C. In some parts of the hospital it was not possible to obtain a water temperature in excess of 58°C even after a 30 minute flush. It was found that the number of *L. pneumophila* recovered from these taps and showers remained undiminished. Consequently, a policy of flushing outlets daily for 15 minutes before patients were allowed to use them was introduced. A year later this policy was modified to a 15 minute weekly flush with water at a temperature between 50 and 58°C. On this new regime, three further cases occurred, but these were attributed to a staff failure in flushing regularly taps in the immediate vicinity of the patients who were affected. There was another failure of the control measures the following year when two patients developed *L. pneumophila* pneumonia 2 weeks after the temperature of the hot water tanks was accidentally lowered to 52°C resulting in tap water temperatures of 36 to 49°C.

In reviewing all the above outbreak control measures, one common theme was found in all the reports. This theme was the particular difficulty encountered in maintaining adequate levels of the bacteriocidal agent, be it heat or chlorine, throughout the water system. This is often a consequence of stagnation due to irregular use or poor flow in the peripheral part of the system. Ciesielski and colleagues (1984), have produced data to suggest that devices such as faucet (tap) aerators which obstruct the flow of water may also encourage the growth of *L. pneumophila*. If faucet aerators or antisplash fittings are found to be heavily colonized by legionellas, then it is obviously sensible to remove such devices which are not essential equipment. The rate of flow in a circulating hot water system may be improved by the installation of an additional pump. Any blind ends arising from the circulating loop should be removed and capped close to the loop. Deadlegs arising from the loop are also unsatisfactory and in many establishments it should be possible to reduce their number. The installation of supplementary terminal heating devices (instantaneous heaters), such as those fitted to many domestic shower units, is another way of tackling the problem. The method adopted by Meenhorst and colleagues (1985) of frequent prolonged flushing of hot water outlets is expensive and liable to human error, as they found in practice.

The variety of strategies adopted in the control of legionellosis is indicative of the lack of comparative studies of this field. Edelstein (1983), has drawn attention to the need for well controlled field studies to provide a scientific basis for decision making. In the absence of such data, the infection control team has to choose methods which have been shown to be effective yet have few disadvantages in terms of hazards to patients, or damage to the hot water system. At present, the best choice appears to be continuous chlorination to 1–2 mg/litre (ppm) of free residual chlorine with the circulating hot water temperature maintained within the range 50–60°C. For the chlorination, either sodium hypochlorite injection units may be used or alternatively, electrolytic chlorination units. Gas chlorination is not recommended because of the capital cost of the equipment and the health risk in the event of a gas leak. Frequent measurements should be made of water temperatures and free residual chlorine levels at taps in various parts of the building, particularly those closest to and furthest from the calorifier. A log should be kept of all results and of quantities of hydrochlorite solution used. All other maintenance procedures on the system should be recorded. As well as these specific measures engineering 'good housekeeping' practices should be followed in the maintenance and operation of the domestic water systems. These are outlined in the section of this chapter which deals with general preventive measures.

Control of outbreaks from cooling water systems

As for hot water systems there have been no well controlled field studies to determine the best means of decontamination and long term control. Consequently, some hospitals have taken the decision to dismantle cooling water systems implicated as sources of legionellosis and replace them with 'air cooled condensers'. In these units, air is blown directly over the condenser coils. Modern units may be as efficient as cooling water systems but the disadvantages of installing them as a control measure can be a high capital cost, running cost and noise production. Some centres have been happy to meet the initial capital cost in the knowledge that the expenditure would provide a permanent long term solution. The running costs appear on face value to be higher than the cost of operating a cooling water system because of greater energy consumption. It is, however, important to take into the equation the additional costs in running a cooling water system which include the costs of chemicals, regular chemical and microbiological tests, water charges and extra maintenance costs resulting from the need for regular draining, cleaning and flushing of the system. In some circumstances, when the cost of electricity is relatively low, the costs of maintaining and operating a cooling water system could well be greater than the costs of an air cooled system, depending on the cooling load. In this respect there is a lack of good comparative data to guide those faced with the choice of implementing control measures.

In general, cooling water systems have not been replaced in the control of outbreaks but chemical treatment of cooling water has generally been accepted as the most cost effective. Most experience in the decontamination of cooling towers or evaporative condensers has been with shock chlorination. To be effective, this chlorination has to be combined with a thorough cleaning of the system including the pipe-work. The principal steps in the procedure will now be described.

The entire system should immediately be shut down. This means that the refrigeration unit or other heat source, fans on the cooling tower or evaporative condenser and the water pumps should be turned off. The cooling tower or evaporative condenser pond should be drained and refilled with fresh water and the blow down valve shut off. Sodium hypochlorite solution or calcium hypochlorite powder should be added in sufficient quantity to achieve a concentration of 50 mg/litre (ppm) of free residual chlorine in the cooling water. The pumps, but not the fans, should be turned on to circulate the cooling water. Acid or alkali should be added to keep the pH within the range 7.2–7.8. It may be necessary to add further hypochlorite at this stage to ensure a minimum concentration of 50 mg/litre (ppm). A large quantity of slime may build up in the cooling water pipework and to remove this organic material it may be necessary to add a chemical dispersant or detergent to the cooling water. It is important that chlorination takes place before and after treatment with dispersant because although the tower fans have been turned off, aerosol may be carried over by natural drafts. Heavy concentrations of *L. pneumophila* in the cooling water may result from treatment with dispersant. At this stage further hypochlorite will probably have to be added to regain a free residual chlorine concentration of 50 mg/litre. The cooling water should continue to recirculate. It is permissible now to allow the free residual chlorine level to fall to 10 mg/litre (ppm), but it should be kept at this minimum value for at least 12 hours. The water pumps should then be turned off and the entire system drained down. Next the cooling tower should be thoroughly cleaned mechanically, or with a steam lance, depending on the shell or packing materials. All sludge and debris in the pond should be removed or flushed away. It is possible that chlorine may not have penetrated completely the organic and inorganic materials that build up in a cooling tower, so it is advisable that the operators undertaking the cleaning should wear biological respirators fitted with high efficiency particulate filters. When the cleaning is completed the entire cooling water system should be refilled and hypochlorite should again be added to achieve 10 mg/litre of free residual chlorine. The water pump should be turned on and further hypochlorite should be added, as necessary, to maintain a minimum chlorine level of 10 mg/litre over a 6 hour period. This should complete the decontamination of the cooling water system. The routine maintenance water treatment programme should be implemented immediately. Such a programme, together with other maintenance procedures including regular cleaning are dealt with in a later section of this chapter which deals with general preventive measures.

Although there have been several studies of the efficacy of various biocides on legionellas, few have been assessed in the field. Cooling water systems are complex ecologies and efficacy demonstrated in the artificial conditions of the laboratory may not be reliably extrapolated to field conditions. Apart from chlorine, one other chemical was shown to be effective in initial decontamination of a cooling tower and control over one year. This chemical, a biodegradable chlorinated phenolic thio-ether, was found to be effective in a small comparative field trial of biocides one summer (Kurtz *et al.*, 1984). The cooling towers which were the source of an outbreak of *L. pneumophila* pneumonia served a compressor house on a power station under construction (Morton *et al.*, 1986). The cooling towers were small capacity units similar to those used for air-conditioning purposes in hospitals, hotels and office blocks. The cooling water was treated with the phenolic thio-ether for a 24 hour period, maintaining a minimum concentration of 500 mg/litre (ppm). The cooling water systems were also treated with a detergent based dispersant and the towers were steamed-cleaned and all debris removed from their packing and ponds. After the system was thoroughly flushed with fresh water it was brought back into operation and weekly dosing of the phenolic thio-ether was incorporated in the regular chemical treatment programme. Subsequent samples from the cooling system, collected on a weekly basis for a year, were negative except on one occasion which followed maintenance work on the cooling water pipe-work. The cooling towers were dismantled at the end of the year when they were no longer required for operational purposes. No new cases of legionnaires' disease have occurred on the site since the cooling water system was decontaminated. Although the phenolic thio-ether was found to be effective in the short term, the data on its efficacy is limited and there is no published data on its performance in the long term.

There is an urgent need for controlled field trials for initial decontamination and long term control. These trials should evaluate not only the efficacy of formulations, but also deleterious effects such as corrosion and overall costs.

Control of outbreaks from other water systems

Experience is very limited in the control of outbreaks from sources other than domestic water systems in hotels and hospitals and cooling water systems. Three recreational whirlpool spas have been associated with legionellosis (Public Health Laboratory Service, 1985; Mangione *et al.*, 1985; Spitalny *et al.*, 1984). At one site the owner took the decision to close down the spas and remove them (Public Health Laboratory Service, 1985) and in the published account of one of the other outbreaks, no description is given of the control measures (Mangione *et al.*, 1985). Continuous chlorination was selected for the other site (Spitalny *et al.*, 1984) and an account of the method has been given by Witherell and colleagues (1984). The whirlpool spa was chlorinated continuously by means of either an automatic sodium hypochlorite solution feed pump or an 'erosion-type' chlorinator. A residual of 1.0 to 3.0 mg/litre (ppm) of free residual chlorine and a pH of 7.2–7.8 were maintained. This treatment resulted in the reduction of *L. pneumophila* to below detectable limits within the first week of treatment and no further cases of legionellosis occurred in association with the pool.

When contaminated respiratory therapy nebulizers have been shown to be the source of infection, then the best solution is to replace them with disposable equipment and use only sterile water. If disposable nebulizers are not available, although ideally they should be used as standard practice in hospitals and clinics, then the implicated apparatus should be dismantled. After thorough cleansing of the equipment and disinfection with sodium hypochlorite solution at 25 ppm for 12 hours, the equipment could be brought back into operation, but only sterile water should be used for the generation of aerosol. As regards water based lubricants, which were implicated as the source of an outbreak of legionellosis in a car assembly plant (Herwaldt *et al.*, 1984), studies are needed to determine the best method of controlling the growth of legionella. It is conventional practice to keep the lubricant within a restricted range of pH, depending on the materials in use, to treat regularly with biocides to inhibit bacterial growth and to circulate the system continuously to prevent separation of water and oil. Whether these measures alone would serve to control the growth of legionella is unclear and deserves study.

General preventive measures

The necessity for the application of control measures to a water system which has been implicated through investigation as a source of legionellosis is clearcut. The indications for preventive measures in buildings which are not known to be associated with legionellosis are less well defined.

A large survey of hospitals, hotels and business premises in Britain, found legionellas to be present in more than half of these establishments, particularly in their domestic hot water and cooling water systems. Engineers should therefore expect to find legionellas in their building services and need not implement drastic control measures if laboratory tests demonstrate the presence of the organism. Indeed, it is generally agreed that routine sampling of domestic water systems and cooling water systems for legionella culture is not helpful as a primary preventive measure. Subtyping of legionellas by monoclonal antibodies has shown that most strains of *L. pneumophila* serogroup 1 found in domestic water and cooling water systems are not of the subtypes which have caused epidemic or sporadic infection in man (Watkins *et al.*, 1985).* Furthermore, whether the organism is found to be present or

* If (a) the work of Watkins *et al.*, 1985 is substantiated and further studies find that *L. pneumophila* serogroup 1 subtypes causing nosocomial outbreaks of legionnaires' disease are present in only a small proportion of hospital water systems and (b) a well validated sub-typing method becomes readily available, then it might be possible to justify the introduction of periodic sampling and, when necessary, disinfection of water systems serving hospital departments (eg. oncology, haemodialysis and organ transplantation units) occupied by patients likely to be particularly susceptible to the infection. Hospital engineers would be ill advised to arrange independently the testing of any building services for legionella. The need for such sampling in hospitals should always be considered jointly by the engineer and the consultant microbiologist.

not, good engineering practices should be followed in the maintenance and operation of all water systems. In Britain, the Department of Health and Social Security in England, the Department of Health and Social Services in Northern Ireland, the Welsh Office and the Scottish Home and Health Department, outlines these good practices in health notices which are issued to health authorities. These health notices give guidance on hospital water systems, but are also suitable for use in hotels, office blocks and other large buildings. The general preventive measures which might be taken in such establishments will now be described in rather more detail than in the health notices. Some additional recommendations are made including advice on design features as well as routine maintenance and operation. The measures which are described are based on the results of studies of building services implicated as sources of legionella infections and from the published results of surveys of water systems. These primary preventive measures are essentially good engineering practices which, if followed, should discourage microbial growth within water systems. It must be emphasized that they have not been evaluated in a controlled fashion and there is a great need for such studies in which attention should be paid to relative costs and potential hazards as well as efficacy.

Domestic water systems in large buildings

Domestic hot water systems in hotels and hospitals have been the most

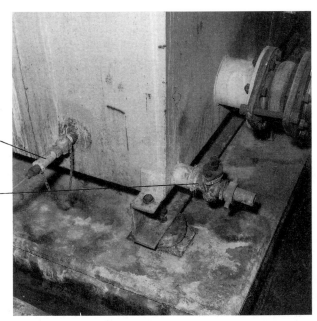

Drain A – A pipe of small diameter which is located in a position that does not permit complete drainage of the tank.

Drain B – A pipe of adequate size which is well positioned at the base of the tank.

Fig. 8.5 A water tank fitted with two drain points.

commonly recognized source of legionellosis in Britain. They have also been implicated in many outbreaks in the USA and Europe (see Table 7.1 and 7.2). Studies of outbreaks have shown that hot water temperatures below 50°C, calorifier design and stagnation within the water system are the principal predisposing factors. There are therefore important lessons for the architect and building services engineer:

(i)   Excess water storage capacity should be avoided to promote an adequate rate of flow through the system.

(ii) Water tanks, if connected in series, should be located on exactly the same level. If the base of one tank is situated even a few millimetres above the others to which it is connected then there will be a differential rate of flow which may lead to relative stagnation and temperature stratification in one of the tanks.

(iii) Water storage tanks should have well fitted covers with lipped edges to prevent entry of dust and other material which could provide a nutritional source for microorganisms. Overflow pipes should be fitted with a fine mesh cover to prevent the entry of birds and vermin.

Water tanks and calorifiers should have a drain which is located on the base or bottom of a side wall to enable complete draining of the tank during cleaning (Fig. 8.5). The drainpipe should be of adequate diameter to enable the flushing away of sludge and other debris.

(iv) Water pipes should be adequately lagged to prevent cold water taking up heat and hot water losing heat; ideally cold water should be stored and circulated at temperatures less than 20°C.

(v)   Calorifiers should be designed in such a way that stratification of water temperature is minimized. In a recent survey legionellas were found less frequently in horizontal than vertical calorifiers, possibly because of temperature stratification, (Bartlett *et al.*, 1986).

(vi) Cul-de-sacs or dead legs should be avoided in the water distribution system. Hot water outlets should always be located as close to the circulating loop as possible.

(vii) Only Water Research Centre approved fixtures and fittings should be incorporated in the system. There is some evidence that certain types of washers may favour the growth of legionellas (Colbourne *et al.*, 1984), others may not (Colbourne and Ashworth, 1986).

In terms of maintenance and operation of domestic water systems, the building services engineer must ensure that all water storage vessels are kept clean and free of debris, by introducing a regular cleaning programme. Particular attention should be paid to calorifiers which have been shown to provide an ecological niche for legionellas. To minimize the build up of sediment, the calorifier drain, if located at the base, should be opened on a regular basis and water flushed through preferably at a time when there is low demand upon the system. An optimum frequency for this procedure has yet to be determined but in the meantime a once monthly schedule would seem to be reasonable. Engineers should take the opportunity to thoroughly clean the internal surfaces of calorifiers and flush away all debris whenever heating coils are required to be inspected. When a calorifier is taken out of operation for a week or more it should be drained down and kept empty until required for further use. If this is not practicable then the drain should be opened prior to use and the vessel flushed through with fresh water. Whenever possible, calorifiers should be allowed to stand overnight after cleaning, draining or flushing, to allow any suspended sediment to settle. Hospital engineers should follow the recommendations of the guidelines issued by the Department of Health and Social Security in England, the Welsh Office and the Scottish Home and Health Department which state that hot water should be stored at a temperature of 60°C and distributed at a temperature not less than 50°C. Because of the risk of scalding, units housing children, the elderly or the mentally handicapped may wish to modify this recommendation until the measure has been demonstrated to be of proven benefit in such establishments. In these units it would be reasonable to circulate the water at temperatures within the range 45–52°C. Whenever water is distributed at temperatures in excess of 55°C warning notices should be placed over every hot water tap and shower, unless there is a thermostatic valve.

Cooling water systems

Studies of outbreaks from cooling towers and evaporative condensers (see Table 7.3) have identified areas in which systems design can be improved:

(i)   Cooling towers or evaporative condensers should not be located in such a position that their drift can readily enter a ventilation system.

(ii)   Drains should be of adequate size and located to allow the pond and all pipe-work to be drained completely.

(iii) To permit adequate cleaning, certain types of cooling tower need to be redesigned for improved accessibility (Bartlett and Pickering, 1983). Modular packs and drift eliminators may help in this respect.

(iv)   Efforts should be made to improve the efficiency of drift eliminators and entrainement devices. Drift is the term used to describe the water droplets in cooling tower and evaporative condenser effluent. Even in well maintained towers the drift loss may reach 0.2 per cent of the circulating cooling water flow rate (Miller, 1979). In poorly designed or inadequately maintained systems the drift loss may be five or six times this amount.

In terms of routine maintenance and operation it is conventional practice to treat cooling waters with corrosion inhibitors, scale inhibitors (except in areas with very soft water) and biocides to prevent 'fouling' or build up of organic material. The reasons for doing this are primarily to maintain the efficiency of heat exchange. A recent survey (Bartlett *et al.*, 1986), found that cooling towers which were corroded or had scaling, fouling, or a build up of debris in the bottom of the pond, tended to yield legionella more commonly than those towers without these factors. The study also found that towers which were cleaned twice a year were significantly less likely to yield legionella than those cleaned only once yearly. It seems that the application of conventional treatment practices for cooling water systems will not only maintain their efficacy but also discourage the growth of legionellas. Although several biocides have looked promising in the laboratory and in a few limited field studies, no single chemical agent has been shown convincingly to be superior to the others, in field trials, for the long term control of legionella in cooling water systems. The choice of biocides and other chemicals will depend on the nature of the water supply and the design of the cooling water system. Engineers are advised to seek the advice of a reputable water treatment company to determine the most suitable regimen for their equipment.

Five per cent or more of the circulating cooling water flow rate may be lost as water vapour through evaporation. As a consequence, organic and inorganic material in the cooling water will be concentrated. To counteract this concentrating effect, a proportion of the cooling water should be regularly discharged to waste and the system topped up with fresh water. This process of 'bleeding' may be carried out automatically or manually. If done automatically, the equipment should be checked regularly to ensure that it is operating correctly. If a system has to be manually blown down then it is advisable to keep a log of this procedure to ensure that it is not overlooked.

In the United Kingdom, health notices issued by the four departments of health recommend that cooling towers and evaporative condensers in hospitals should be cleaned at least twice yearly. Perhaps engineers should make regular, say monthly, inspections of evaporative coolers and implement cooling whenever there is evidence of organic fouling with slime or algae. To protect the operators it is advisable that the cooling water be chlorinated prior to cleaning; it is recommended that the cooling water be chlorinated and circulated for 4 hours, an arbitrary but practical period, maintaining a minimum level of free residual chlorine of 5 mg/litre (ppm). If there is a bypass loop the chlorinated water should be circulated through it, ideally simultaneously with circulation through the pond (see Fig. 8.4). If necessary a chemical dispersant should be used to clear fouling in the cooling water pipe-work. The cooling tower or evaporative condenser's internal shell, packing material and pond should be thoroughly cleansed mechanically or by means of a steam lance, depending on the construction materials. The equipment should be thoroughly flushed with fresh water to remove sediment and other debris.

When the flushings are clear, the system should be topped up with fresh water and the routine chemical treatment regimen implemented immediately. At the time of cleaning the drift eliminators should be inspected and if found to be damaged should be repaired or replaced. Engineers should ensure that a log is kept of chemical treatments and the periodic inspection and clean.

Respiratory therapy equipment and other humidification systems

Humidifiers and nebulizers used for respiratory therapy are often neglected pieces of equipment. These are commonly used by patients with underlying lung disease who may be at increased risk of infection. Not infrequently, organic growth may occur in this equipment and several of the micro-organisms responsible may cause opportunistic infection in patients. It is important, therefore, that the equipment is thoroughly cleaned on a regular basis with a sodium hypochlorite solution and detergent. Removable parts should be soaked in a dilute sodium hypochlorite solution (5 mg/litre (ppm) free residual chlorine) for 6 hours. Thereafter, the equipment should be thoroughly rinsed. Ideally disposable nebulizers should be used. Only sterile water should be used in equipment designed for respiratory therapy.

Larger scale humidification equipment and recirculating air wash systems found in some ventilation systems have not been found to be sources of legionellosis. The reason for this is open to speculation but temperature may be an important factor. In general, the temperatures found in such systems be they of spinning disc, pan heater or spray design, are generally not within the range which favours the rapid growth of legionella. Dry steam injection devices do not present problems with microbial growth unless there is pooling of condensate within the ventilation system.

The recirculating spray type humidifiers have been associated with a disease called humidifier fever. This was first described in the annual report of HM Inspector of Factories (1969) and several outbreaks have been documented since then. This is probably a hypersensitivity reaction to certain microorganisms which can grow in humidifiers. No evidence of legionella infection has been found in serum specimens collected from cases during the investigation of outbreaks. As for cooling water systems, a regular cleaning programme is perhaps the most important preventive measure which can be applied. Whenever practicable the water supply to such units should be derived directly from a rising main. An adequate blow down is essential to prevent a build up in the concentration of organic and inorganic materials. In some industrial settings, particularly when there is a high level of cellulose dust in the building, as found in some printing works, regular cleaning alone has not been sufficient to prevent organic growth within the system. Under these circumstances, a different method of humidification has been introduced or alternatively regular water treatment instituted with biocides (Bartlett and Pickering, 1983). The effects of long term exposure to low levels of such chemicals in man are unknown.

Spas and whirlpools

Spas and whirlpools in which water is recirculated, but not changed after each use, present particular problems for the maintenance of water quality. It is general practice to change the water quite infrequently because of the cost of reheating the water and chemical treatment. Several hundred people may use a spa bath between complete water changes, although the circulating water volume may be no more than five times that of a domestic bath tub. This results in a considerable organic load within the system which may be compounded by air and water jets which encourage the loss of skin scales and other body materials. The water in these recreational baths is heated to between 30 and 42°C and with these comfortable temperatures some individuals may spend several hours in a spa at any one time. All these factors tend to encourage microbial growth within the bath water. Preventive chemical treatment is particularly difficult because of the high organic load and a fluctuating pH. Jones and Bartlett (1985), have suggested that adequate water quality can only be achieved in heavily used public and commercial spas and whirlpools by regular draining of the entire system, and replenishment with fresh water, continuous rather than intermittent dosing with biocides and a restriction of the number of bathers using the pool each day. Chlorination and bromination are likely to be the most effective and acceptable methods for controlling the growth of legionella in spas . There is, however, a very great need for a well controlled study of different chemical treatment regimens to decide which is the most effective in the long term. The authors feel it is essential that a daily log is kept of the quantities of chemicals used in treatment as well as pH, free residual halogen or any other test results. In heavily used and public pools it will be advisable, as a minimum, to have testing before the pool is brought into use for the day and thereafter at 2 hourly intervals. The log of treatment and tests should be available for inspection by local authority environmental health officers. In Britain the Swimming Pool and Allied Trades Association (SPATA), have recently issued comprehensive guidelines on the installation and maintenance of commercial spa pools. If outbreaks of legionellosis and other infections such as those caused by *Pseudomonas aeruginosa*, continue to occur despite the considerable publicity devoted to them and the availability of the SPATA guidelines, then local authorities should consider enacting legislation which will require commercial and public pools to be registered. Regular inspections should then be made by environmental health officers who may wish to take samples occasionally for routine water microbiology as well as to check the log.

References

Baird, I.M., Potts, W., Smiley, J. *et al.* (1984). Control of endemic nosocomial legionellosis by hyperchlorination of potable water. In *Legionella. Proceedings of the 2nd International Symposium; Washington, DC.*, p. 333. Edited by Thornsberry, C., Balows, A. Feeley, J.C. and Jakubowski, W.J. American Society for Microbiology, Washington.

Bartlett, C.L.R. and Bibby, L.F. (1983). Epidemic Legionellosis in England and Wales 1979-1982. *Zentralblatt fur Bakteriologie, Parasitenkunde, Infektionskrankheiten und Hygiene I. Abteilung: Originale* A **255**, 64-70.

Bartlett, C.L.R., Dennis, P.J.L., Harper, D. *et al.* (1986). Legionella in plumbing systems. Submitted for publication.

Bartlett, C.L.R. and Pickering, C.A.C. (1983). Medical Aspects of Air Conditioning and Other Building Services. In *Air Conditioning System Design for Building*. Edited by A.F.C. Sherratt. McGraw Hill, London.

Bartlett, C.L.R., Swann, R.A., Canada Royo, C.L. *et al.* (1984). Recurrent Legionnaires' disease from a hotel water system. In *Legionella. Proceedings of the 2nd International Symposium; Washington, DC.*, pp. 237-9. Edited by Thornsberry, C., Balows, A., Feeley J.C. and Jakubowski, W.J. American Society for Microbiology, Washington.

Best, M., Stout, J., Muder, R.R. *et al.* (1983). Legionellaceae in the hospital water supply. *Lancet* **ii**, 307-10.

British Thoracic Society Research Committee. (1986). Community-acquired pneumonia in adults in British hospitals in 1982-3: A BTS/PHLS survey of aetiology, mortality, prerequisite factors and outcome. *QJM* In press.

Ciesielski, C.A., Blaser, M.J., Laforce, M. *et al*. (1984). Role of stagnation and obstruction of water flow in isolation of *Legionella pneumophila* from hospital plumbing. In *Legionella. Proceedings of the 2nd International Symposium; Washington DC.*, pp. 307–9. Edited by Thornsberry, C., Balows, A., Feeley J.C. and Jakubowski, W.J. American Society for Microbiology, Washington.

Colbourne, J.S. and Ashworth, J. (1986). Rubbers, water and legionella. *Lancet* 2, 583.

Colbourne, J.S., Pratt, D.J., Smith, M.G. *et al*. (1984). The role of water fittings as sources of *Legionella pneumophila* in a hospital's plumbing system. *Lancet* 1, 210–13.

Department of the Environment, Department of Health and Social Security, Public Health Laboratory Service. (1982). *The Bacteriological Examination of Drinking Water Supplies*. Reports on Public Health and Medical Subjects **No. 71** Methods for the Examination of Waters and Associated Materials.

Dondero, T.J., Rendtorff, R.C., Mallison, G.F. *et al*. (1980). An outbreak of Legionnaires' disease associated with a contaminated air conditioning cooling tower. *N Engl J Med* **302**, 365–70.

Edelstein, P.H. (1983). What to do about legionella? *JAMA* **249**, 3214–15.

Fisher-Hoch, S.P., Bartlett, C.L.R., Tobin, J.O'H. *et al*. (1981). Investigation and control of an outbreak of Legionnaires' disease in a district general hospital. *Lancet* **1**, 932–6.

Fisher-Hoch, S.P., Smith, M.G., Colbourne, J.S. (1982). *Legionella pneumophila* in hospital hot water cylinders. *Lancet* **i**, 1073.

Fraser, D.W., Tsai, T.R., Orenstein, W. *et al*. (1977). Legionnaires' disease: description of an epidemic of pneumonia. *N Engl J Med* **297**, 1189–97.

Friedman, G.D. (1974). *Primer of Epidemiology*. McGraw Hill, London.

Galbraith, N.S. (1982). *Communicable Disease Surveillance*. Edited by A. Smith Churchill Livingstone.

Helms, C.M., Massanari, R.M., Zeitler, R. *et al*. (1983). Legionnaires' disease associated with a hospital water system: a cluster of 24 nosocomial cases. *Ann Intern Med* **99**, 172–8.

Herwaldt, L.A., Gorman, G.W., McGrath, T. *et al*. (1984). A new Legionella species, *Legionella feeleii* species nova, causes Pontiac fever in an automobile plant. *Ann Intern Med* **100**, 333–8.

Jones, F. and Bartlett, C.L.R. (1985). Infections associated with whirlpools and spas. *J Appl Bacteriol*. 61S–66S.

Kurtz, J.B., Bartlett, C.L.R., Tillett, H.E. *et al*. (1984). Field trial of biocides in the control of *Legionella pneumophila* in cooling water systems. In *Legionella. Proceedings of the 2nd International Symposium; Washington, DC.*, pp. 340–42. Edited by Thornsberry, C., Balows, A., Feeley J.C. and Jakubowski, W.J. American Society of Microbiology, Washington.

Langmuir, A.D. (1963). The surveillance of communicable diseases of national importance. *N Engl J Med* **268**, 82–192.

Mangione, E.J., Remis, R.S., Tait, K.A. *et al*., (1985). An outbreak of Pontiac fever related to whirlpool use, Michigan 1982. *JAMA*. **253**, 535–9.

Massanari, R.M., Helms, C., Zeitler, R. *et al*. (1984). Continuous hyperchlorination of a potable water system for control of nosocomial *Legionella pneumophila* infections. In *Legionella. Proceedings of the 2nd International Symposium; Washington, DC.*, pp. 334–6. Edited by Thornsberry, C., Balows, A., Feeley, J.C. and Jakubowski, W.J. American Society for Microbiology, Washington.

Meenhorst. P.L., Reingold, A.L., Groothuis, D.G. *et al*. (1985). Water-related nosocomial pneumonia caused by *Legionella pneumophila* serogroup 1 and 10. *J Infect Dis* **152**, 356–63.

Miller, R.P. (1979). Cooling towers and evaporative condensers. *Ann Intern Med* **90**, 667–70.

Morton, S., Bartlett, C.L.R., Bibby, L.F. *et al.* (1986). An outbreak of legionnaires' disease from a cooling water system in a power station. *Br J Indust Med* **43**, 630–35.

Neill, M.A., Gorman, G.F., Gibert, C. *et al.* (1985). Nosocomial legionellosis, Paris, France. *Am J Med* **78**, 581–8.

Palmer, S.R., Zamiri, I., Ribeiro, C.D. *et al.* Legionnaires' disease cluster and reduction in hospital hot water temperatures. *Br Med J* **292**, 1494–5.

Public Health Laboratory Service Communicable Disease Surveillance Centre. (1985). CDR 85/50.

Public Health Laboratory Service. (1986). Report on a collaborative study of legionella species in water systems 1981–1985. Unpublished.

Rudin, J. and Wing, E.J. (1984). An ongoing outbreak of *Legionella micdadei*. In *Legionella. Proceedings of the 2nd International Symposium, Washington, DC.*, pp. 227–9. Edited by Thornsberry, C., Balows, A., Feeley, J.C. and Jakubowski, W.J. American Society for Microbiology, Washington.

Shands, K.N., Ho, J.L., Meyer, R.D. (1985). Potable water as a source of Legionnaires' disease. *JAMA* **253**, 1412–16.

Spitalny, K.C., Vogt, R.L., Orciari, L.A. *et al.* (1984). Pontiac fever associated with a whirlpool spa. *Am J Epidemiol* **120**, 809–17.

Tobin, J.O'H., Dunhill, M.S., French, M. *et al.* (1980). Legionnaires' disease in a transplant unit: isolation of the causative agent from shower baths. *Lancet* **ii**, 118–21.

Tobin, J.O'H., Bartlett, C.L.R., Waitkins, S.A. *et al.* (1981). Legionnaires' disease: Further evidence to implicate water storage and distribution systems as sources. *Br Med J* **282**, 573.

Watkins, I.D., Tobin, J.O.H., Dennis, P.J. *et al.* (1985). *Legionella pneumophila* serogroup 1 subgrouping by monoclonal antibodies – an epidemiological tool. *J Hyg Camb.* **95**, 211–16.

Witherell, L.E., Orciari, L.A., Spitalny, K.C. *et al.* (1984). Disinfection of *Legionella pneumophila* – contaminated whirlpool spas. In *Legionella. Proceedings of the 2nd International Symposium; Washington, DC.*, pp. 336–7. Edited by Thornsberry, C., Balows, A., Feeley, J.C. and Jakubowski, W.J. American Society for Microbiology, Washington.

Appendix: The Environmental Reservoir of Legionella, Potential Sources and Routes of Infection

In order to make this work as up to date as possible at the time of publication, this appendix has been added to include a balanced review of issues which have been raised recently on sources and modes of transmission.

The *Legionellaceae* have been found in numerous natural aquatic habitats and man-made water systems. *L. pneumophila* has been isolated from lakes, rivers, streams and mud (Fliermans *et al.*, 1979, 1981; Morris *et al.*, 1979) and even collections of rain water in rain forests in Puerto Rico (Ortiz-Roque and Hazen, 1982). Surveys in several countries have shown that plumbing systems in buildings are commonly colonized by *L. pneumophila* and occasionally by other species (Arnow *et al.*, 1985; Bartlett *et al.*, 1983, 1986; Dennis *et al.*, 1982; Desplaces *et al.*, 1984; Joly *et al.*, 1985; Peel *et al.*, 1985; Tobin *et al.*, 1981a, 1986; Wadowsky *et al.*, 1982). Legionellas have also been found frequently in cooling water systems used for air-conditioning or industrial purposes (Bartlett *et al.*, 1986; Christensen *et al.*, 1984; Desplaces *et al.*, 1984; Kurtz *et al.*, 1982; Soloman *et al.*, 1984, Witherell *et al.*, 1984). There is good epidemiological evidence that hot water systems, cooling water systems and several other specific types of water system serve as sources of legionellosis (see Chapter 7). Other water systems which release water droplets into the air might be considered as potential sources of infection.

Water is used widely in many industrial processes and it is surprising that some such 'process' waters have not been shown to serve as sources of legionellosis. Unexplained outbreaks in industry have been reported, however, one of which occurred as early as 1957 in a meat packing plant in Austin, USA (Osterholm *et al.*, 1983). In another incident, there is indirect evidence that stored water used for cleaning drilling equipment on an oil rig may have been responsible for at least one case of legionnaires' disease (Castellani-Pastoris *et al.*, 1986).

Many other types of water system, such as those used with high speed dental drills, fountains, fire sprinklers and car washes, are known to harbour the organism but have not been reported to have caused outbreaks of legionellosis. This may be because one or more links in the chain of causation are absent (see Chapter 7, pp. 90). There may be a lack of 'amplification' factors, the most important of which is a suitable temperature. Although *L. pneumophila* has been isolated from water at temperatures ranging from 5.7° to 63°C (Fliermans *et al.*, 1981), it probably only multiplies actively from about 20° to 45°C. The organism is quite heat tolerant, but it begins to die at 50°C and at 58°C there is a 90 per cent loss every 6 minutes (Dennis *et al.*, 1984). At 60°C there is a 90 per cent kill every 2 minutes (Dennis P.J.L.: personal communication). In a recent survey of 176 establishments, including hospitals, hotels and business premises, legionellas were isolated only rarely from hot water systems at temperatures below 40°C or above 60°C (Bartlett *et al.*, 1986). Another link in the chain which may be missing is the ability to disseminate the organism. The system may release into the air mainly large water droplets so that a small particle aerosol is not generated. Infection by means of the respiratory route will not occur unless sufficient numbers of viable organisms are present in droplets or droplet nuclei which are small enough ($< 5\mu$) to be inhaled.

One other explanation for the lack of good evidence to implicate the water systems mentioned above could be that existing surveillance methods lack sensitivity. It is likely, however, that if any of these water systems were important sources of legionella infection, then the evidence would have been produced by now.

It has been proposed that dust may serve as a vehicle in the transmission of legionellosis. This was first suggested by Thacker and colleagues (1978), who reported an outbreak of pneumonia which occurred in 1965 and was unsolved at the time but was shown in 1977 to be caused by *L. pneumophila*. The outbreak took place in Washington, USA in a psychiatric hospital and affected 81 patients. Epidemiological studies showed a higher risk of illness among persons sleeping by open windows and having access to the grounds. There was also a temporal relationship with excavation work in the hospital grounds where a water-sprinkler system was being installed; two clusters followed the closure of two excavation sites. The investigators concluded that the aetiological agent may have resided in the soil and that airborne transmission from the excavation sites took place. In the light of our present knowledge of legionellosis, the most plausible explanation is that the water-sprinkler systems served as the source. It is likely that the sprinklers will have been tested at the time of closure of the sites and that infections resulted from the inhalation of small water droplets or droplet nuclei containing *L. pneumophila*.

Not infrequently, excavation work has been reported in association with outbreaks of legionellosis, particularly when cooling water systems have been implicated as sources. This was so in the original outbreak of Pontiac fever (Glick *et al.*, 1978) and in an outbreak of legionnaires' disease in San Francisco in 1980 (Conwill *et al.*, 1982). An association with building work was also reported in a nosocomial outbreak in which a hot water system was considered to be the source (Parry *et al.*, 1985). On this occasion *L. bozemanii*, the aetiological agent, was isolated from the water system and soil on the excavation site nearby. The significance of the link with excavation sites is obscure and may be merely coincidental, but perhaps dust may provide a source of nutrition to legionella in water systems, particularly cooling waters, and occasionally may be responsible for seeding the system.

Other routes of infection

Woo and colleagues (1986) have recently questioned the mode of transmission of legionellosis in hospitals. They undertook experiments to evaluate the ability of showers, humidifiers and respiratory equipment to generate aerosols containing *L. pneumophila*. They were unable to detect such aerosols from showers but they found that portable humidifiers were able to produce them readily. They also found that rinsing of ventilation bags with tap water led to the isolation of *L. pneumophila* on culture plates after the bags were squeezed. In earlier work, Yu and colleagues (1981), had produced indirect evidence that aspiration of contaminated water could be a route of infection for *L. pneumophila*. Muder and colleagues (1982), in a prospective study of pneumonia found that patients with legionnaires' disease were significantly more likely than others to have undergone endotracheal intubation. The weight of evidence is sufficient to advise staff in intensive care units to avoid rinsing ventilation bag adaptors and tubing with tap water, a practice which is more widespread in some countries than others.

Perhaps too much emphasis has been placed on showering as a mode of transmission but it should not be dismissed altogether. Other experimental work has demonstrated that showers can generate aerosols of *L. pneumophila* (Dennis *et al.*, 1984; Bollin *et al.*, 1985). Furthermore, the lack of direct epidemiological evidence may be explained by the technical problems involved in study design (see Chapter 7, p. 101). Without doubt, insufficient attention has been paid to taps (faucets) as generators of aerosols of *L. pneumophila*. There is good experimental evidence that airborne dissemination of the organism can take place from both hand basins and bath taps as a result of surface impaction (Dennis P.J.L.: personal communication). There are also documented outbreaks of legionnaires' disease from hot water systems in hotels in which persons affected had not had showers but had had conventional baths (Bartlett *et al.*, 1984; Tobin *et al.*, 1981b). This mode of transmission is likely to exist also in hospitals (Fisher-Hoch *et al.*, 1981).

When considering all the evidence, inhalation appears to be the most important route of infection but aspiration of the organism during certain medical and nursing procedures may occasionally result in legionella pneumonia. In considering the possibility of endogenous nosocomial infection, Bridge and Edelstein (1983) were unable to find oropharyngeal colonization with *L. pneumophila* in any of 186 volunteers.

Another possible mechanism of infection was suggested in the investigation of nosocomial legionnaires' disease in a hospital in Connecticut, USA. Jones and colleagues (1984), reported a significant association with antacid use, steroid therapy and use of nebulizers. Among patients receiving steroids, antacid use greatly increased the risk of developing legionnaires' disease. It is difficult to draw firm conclusions from this study because of the confounding effect of nebulizer use. The authors put forward the hypothesis that *L. pneumophila* may be ingested and then aspirated into the lungs, a neutral gastric pH facilitating the process. Another explanation is that the gut wall may serve as a portal of entry with spread to the lungs through the bloodstream. Dournon and colleagues (1982), concluded that this was the probable mechanism of infection in a case of legionnaires' disease with *L. pneumophila* peritonitis. The absence of similar reports suggests that if this mode of transmission does take place then it does so only rarely. This route of infection has not been reported in animals, nor have the conjunctivae been shown to serve as a portal of entry.

One final route of infection needs to be considered – parenteral inoculation – although the evidence to suggest it is scanty. There is one report of a patient who developed an *L. pneumophila* abscess at a haemodialysis fistula site (Kalweit *et al.*, 1982) and another of a woman who developed a *L. micdadei* skin abscess on her leg (Ampel *et al.*, 1985). In both instances it was thought that bacteraemic seeding via the lungs was the probable explanation rather than direct inoculation. Finally, there is a report of a patient in whom a hip wound became infected with *L. pneumophila* and *Pseudomonas aeruginosa* following bathing in a contaminated whirlpool spa (Brabender *et al.*, 1983).

References

Ampel, N.M., Ruben, F.L. and Norden, C.W. (1985). Cutaneous abscess caused by *Legionella micdadei* in an immunosuppressed patient. *Ann Intern Med* **102**, 630–33.

Arnow, P.M., Weil, D. and Para, M.F. (1985). Prevalence and significance of *Legionella pneumophila* contamination of residential hot-tap water systems. *J Infect Dis* **152**, 145–51.

Bartlett, C.L.R., Dennis, P.J.L., Harper, D. *et al.* (1986). Legionella in plumbing systems. Submitted for publication.

Bartlett, C.L.R., Kurtz, J.B., Hutchinson, J.G.P. *et al.* (1983). Legionella in hospital and hotel water supplies. *Lancet* **ii**, 1315.

Bartlett, C.L.R., Swann, R.A., Canada Royo, C.L. *et al.* (1984). Recurrent Legionnaires' disease from a hotel water system. In *Legionella. Proceedings of the 2nd International Symposium: Washington, D.C.*, pp. 210–15. Edited by Thornsberry, C., Barlows, A., Feeley, J.C. and Jakubowski, W. American Society for Microbiology Washington.

Bollin, G.E., Plouffe, J.F., Para, M.F. *et al.* (1985). Difference in virulence of environmental isolates of *Legionella pneumophila*. *J Clin Microbiol* **21**, 674–7.

Brabender, W., Hinthorn, D.R., Asher, M. *et al.* (1983). *Legionella pneumophila* wound infection. *JAMA* **250**, 3091–2.

Bridge, J.A. and Edelstein, P.H. (1983). Oropharyngeal colonization with *Legionella pneumophila*. *J Clin Microbiol* **18**, 1108–12.

Castellani-Pastoris, M., Greco, D., Vassello, A. *et al.* (1986). Legionnaires' disease on an oil drilling platform in the Mediterranean Sea: a case report. Submitted for publication.

Christensen, S.W., Tyndall, R.L., Soloman, J.A. *et al.* (1984). Patterns of *Legionella spp.* Infectivity in power plant environments and implications for control. In *Legionella: Proceedings of the 2nd International Symposium: Washington, D.C.*, pp. 313–5. Edited by Thornsberry, C., Balows, A., Feeley, J.C. and Jakubowski, W. American Society for Microbiology, Washington.

Conwill, D.E., Benson Werner, S., Dritz, S.K. *et al.* (1982). Legionellosis, the 1980 San Francisco outbreak. *Am Rev Infect Dis* **126**, 666–9.

Dennis, P.J., Green, D and Jones, B.P.C. (1984). A note on the temperature tolerance of *Legionella*. *J Appl Bacteriol* **56**, 349–50.

Dennis, P.J.L., Taylor, L.A., Fitzgeorge, R.B. *et al.* (1982). *Legionella pneumophila* in water plumbing systems. *Lancet* **i**, 949–51.

Dennis, P.J.L., Wright, A.E., Rutter, D.A. *et al.* (1984). *Legionella pneumophila* in aerosols from shower baths. *J Hyg (Camb)* **93**, 349–53.

Desplaces, N., Bure, A. and Dournon, E. (1984). *Legionella spp.* in environmental water samples in Paris. In *Legionella. Proceedings of the 2nd International Symposium: Washington, D.C.*, pp. 320–21. Edited by Thornsberry, C., Balows, A., Feeley, J.C. and Jakubowski, W. American Society for Microbiology, Washington.

Dournon, E., Bure, A., Kemeny, J.L. *et al.* (1982). *Legionella pneumophila* peritonitis. *Lancet* **i**, 1363.

Fisher-Hoch, S.P., Bartlett, C.L.R., Harper, G.J. (1981). Legionnaire's disease at Kingston Hospital. *Lancet* **i**, 1154.

Fliermans, C.B., Cherry, W.B., Orrison, L.H. *et al.* (1979). Isolation of *Legionella pneumophila* from non epidemic-related aquatic habitats. *Appl Environ Microbiol* **37**, 1239–42.

Fliermans, C.B., Cherry, W.B., Orrison, L.H. *et al.* (1981). Ecological distribution of *Legionella pneumophila*. *Appl Environ Microbiol* **41**, 9–16.

Glick, T.H., Gregg, M.B., Berman, B. *et al.* (1978). Pontiac fever: an epidemic of unknown etiology in a health department: I. clinical and epidemiologic aspects. *Am J Epidemiol* **107**, 149–160.

Joly, J.R., Dewailly, E., Bernard, L. *et al.* (1985). Legionella and domestic water heaters in the Quebec City Area. *Can Med Assoc J* **132**, 160.

Jones, E., Checko, P., Dalton, A. *et al.* (1984). Nosocomial Legionnaires' disease associated wtih exposure to respiratory therapy equipment, Connecticut. In *Legionella. Proceedings of the 2nd International Symposium: Washington, D.C.*, pp. 225–7. Edited by Thornsberry, C., Balows, A., Feeley, J.C. and Jakubowski, W. American Society for Microbiology, Washington.

Kalweit, W.H., Winn, W.C., Rocco, T.A. *et al.* (1982). Hemodialysis Fistula infections caused by *Legionella pneumophila*. *Ann Intern Med* **96**, 173–5.

Morris, G.K., Patton, C.M., Feeley, J.C. *et al.* (1979). Isolation of the Legionnaires' disease bacterium from environmental samples. *Ann Intern Med* **90**, 664–6.

Muder, R.R., Yu, V.L., McClure, J.K. *et al.* (1983). Nosocomial Legionnaires' disease uncovered in a prospective pneumonia study. *JAMA* **249**, 3184–8.

Ortiz-Roque and Hazen. (1982). Abstract of the Annual Meeting. American Society for Microbiology, **180**.

Osterholm, M.T., Chin, T.D.Y., Osborne, D.O. *et al.* (1983). A 1957 outbreak of Legionnaires' disease associated with a meat packing plant. *Am J Epidemiol* **117**, 60–67.

Parry, M.F., Stampleman, L., Hutchinson, J.H. *et al.* (1985). Waterborne *Legionella bozemanii* and nosocomial pneumonia in immunosuppressed patients. *Ann Intern Med* **103**, 205–210.

Peel, M.M., Calwell, J.M., Christopher, P.J. *et al.* (1985). *Legionella pneumophila* and water temperatures in Australian hospitals. *Aust NZ J Med* **15**, 38–41.

Soloman, J.A., Christensen, S.W., Tyndall, R.L. *et al.* (1984). Distribution of *Legionella pneumophila* in power plant environments. In *Legionella. Proceedings of the 2nd International Symposium: Washington, D.C.*, pp. 309–11. Edited by Thornsberry, C., Balows, A., Feeley, J.C. and Jakubowski, W. American Society for Microbiology, Washington.

Thacker, S.B., Bennett, J.V., Tsai, T.F. *et al.* (1978). An outbreak in 1965 of severe respiratory illness caused by the Legionnaires' disease bacterium. *J. Infect Dis* **138**, 512–9.

Tobin, R.S., Ewan, P., Walsh, K. *et al.* (1986). A survey of *Legionella pneumophila* in water in 12 Canadian cities. *Wat Res* **20**, 495–501.

Tobin, J.O'H, Swann, R.A. and Bartlett, C.L.R. (1981a). Isolation of *Legionella pneumophila* from water systems: methods and preliminary results. *Brit Med J* **282**, 515–7.

Tobin, J.O'H., Bartlett, C.L.R., Waitkins, S.A. *et al.* (1981b). Legionnaires' disease: further evidence to implicate water storage and distribution systems as sources. *Brit Med J* **282**, 573.

Wadowsky, R.M., Yee, R.B., Mezmar, L. *et al.* (1982). Hot water systems as sources of *Legionella pneumophila* in hospital and nonhospital plumbing fixtures. *Appl Environ Microbiol* **43**, 1104–10.

Witherell, L.E., Novick, L.F., Stone, K.M. *et al.* (1984). *Legionella pneumophila* in Vermont Cooling Towers. In *Legionella. Proceedings of the 2nd International Symposium: Washington, D.C.*, pp. 315–6. Edited by Thornsberry, C., Balows, A., Feeley, J.C. and Jakubowski, W. American Society for Microbiology, Washington.

Woo, A.H., Yu, V.L. and Goetz, A. (1986). Potential In-hospital modes of transmission of *Legionella pneumophila*. *Amer J Med* **80**, 567–73.

Yu, V.L., Stout, J., and Zuravleff, J.J. (1981). Aspiration of contaminated water may be a mode of transmission for *Legionella pneumophila*. Abstract **297**, Intersci Conf Antimicrob Agents Chemother, Chicago.

Index

Index